Veterinary Fluid Therapy

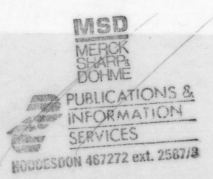

Veterinary Fluid Therapy

A.R. Michell BSc, BVetMed, PhD, MRCVS, FRSA

R.J. Bywater BVM&S, MSc, PhD, MRCVS

K.W. Clarke MA, VetMB, DVetMed, MRCVS, DVA

L.W. Hall MA, BSc, PhD, MRCVS, DVA

A.E. Waterman BVSc, PhD, MRCVS, DVA

Blackwell Scientific Publications

OXFORD LONDON EDINBURGH

BOSTON MELBOURNE

© 1989 by
Blackwell Scientific Publications
Editorial offices:
Osney Mead, Oxford OX2 0EL
  (*Orders*: Tel. 0865 240201)
8 John Street, London WC1N 2ES
23 Ainslie Place, Edinburgh EH3 6AJ
3 Cambridge Center, Suite 208
  Cambridge, Massachusetts 02142, USA
107 Barry Street, Carlton
  Victoria 3053, Australia

First published 1989

Set by Setrite Typesetters,
Hong Kong; printed and bound
in Great Britain by
Mackays of Chatham PLC

DISTRIBUTORS

USA
  Year Book Medical Publishers
  200 North LaSalle Street
  Chicago, Illinois 60601
  (*Orders*: Tel. 312 726-9733)

Canada
  The C.V. Mosby Company
  5240 Finch Avenue East
  Scarborough, Ontario
  (*Orders*: Tel. 416 298-1588)

Australia
  Blackwell Scientific Publications
  (Australia) Pty Ltd
  107 Barry Street
  Carlton, Victoria 3053
  (*Orders*: Tel. (03) 347-0300)

British Library
Cataloguing in Publication Data

Veterinary fluid therapy
  1. Veterinary medicine. Fluid
  therapy
  I. Michell, A.R.
  636.089'539

ISBN 0-632-01407-5

'Doctor Christopher Wren did propose in the University of Oxford ... to that noble benefactor of experimental philosophy Mr Robert Boyle ... that he thought he could easily contrive a way to convey any liquid thing immediately into the mass of the blood by making ligatures on the veins and opening them on the side of the ligature towards the heart, and by putting into them slender syringes or quills, fastened to bladders containing the matter to be injected: performing that operation upon pretty big and lean dogs, that the vessels might be large enough and easily accessible.

'He was the first author of the noble anatomical experiment of injecting liquor into the veins of animals ... hence arose many new experiments and chiefly that of transfusing blood which the Society has prosecuted in sundry instances that will probably end in extraordinary success.'

Documents of the Royal Society
relating to Wren's experiments of 1656 and cited by his son in
'Parentalia: Memoirs of the Family of the Wrens'
by Christopher Wren; published by Stephen Wren,
London MDCCL (pp. 227−8)

Contents

Colour plates 1—4 between pages 142 and 143

List of authors

A.R. Michell BSc, BVetMed, PhD, MRCVS, FRSA
Reader in Experimental Veterinary Medicine, Royal Veterinary College, University of London

R.J. Bywater BVM&S, MSc, PhD, MRCVS
Head of Pharmacology, Beecham Group Ltd, Animal Health Research Centre, Tadworth

K.W. Clarke MA, VetMB, DVetMed, MRCVS, DVA
Senior Lecturer, Department of Surgery, Royal Veterinary College, University of London

L.W. Hall MA, BSc, PhD, MRCVS, DVA
Reader in Comparative Anaesthesia, Department of Clinical Veterinary Medicine (Surgery Division), University of Cambridge

A.E. Waterman BVSc, PhD, MRCVS, DVA
Lecturer, Department of Veterinary Surgery, University of Bristol School of Veterinary Science

Introduction

This book is, in the truest sense, the product of joint authorship. Every chapter has been discussed in detail by each author and modified accordingly; most chapters were initially written by more than one member of the group. Its object is to begin by persuading the reader that the principles of fluid therapy are rational and intelligible, and to end by giving the reader confidence that it is feasible to apply these principles without too much practical difficulty.

The literature on veterinary fluid therapy does not contain sufficient properly designed clinical trials to allow statements of 'right' and 'wrong'. Within the group, however, the range of expertise has been sufficient, we hope, to be able to blend sound theory, direct experience, and the published experience of others. This is not a scholarly work of reference; the primary aims are clarity and applicability. The use of references does not aim to be comprehensive — nevertheless it is intended that the references provide sufficient access to the literature to substantiate the views expressed. Where we have cited our own work, it is frequently to provide access to a more detailed bibliography.

What is fluid therapy? Obviously it mainly comprises the provision of water and simple solutes, orally or parenterally, in adequate quantities to correct abnormalities of plasma volume, plasma composition or underlying cell deficits. The crucial solutes are provided directly or in the form of simple precursors; the mainstream materials do not act via pharmacological properties, i.e. relatively potent effects on tissue receptors or organ functions. Nevertheless, pharmacological agents such as corticosteroids, antibiotics and diuretics can play an important ancillary role in conditions requiring fluid therapy. The boundaries are not quite so clear-cut, however; for example, the use of hypertonic saline in small volumes for the treatment of shock (Chapter 4) reflects pharmacological effects rather than simple volume replacement. The treatment of milk fever or hypomagnesaemia could fall within the scope of fluid therapy. So could the treatment of bovine or ovine acetonaemia or therapy for hypothermia and hypoglycaemia in lambs. Here the decisions to include or exclude under 'fluid therapy' become much more arbitrary. Some texts on fluid therapy certainly include disturbances of divalent ion metabolism. Moreover there are important interactions between, for example, magnesium and potassium disturbances or between hypercalcaemia and polyuria. Nevertheless, in general, these metabolic disorders present relatively discrete entities with a pathogenesis, prevention and treatment largely independent of the main considerations of fluid therapy. They are, therefore, omitted from this book. Other disorders such as diabetes mellitus, myoglobinuria, acute pancreatitis or hepatic failure, produce not only metabolic disturbances but effects on circulating volume, plasma sodium, ICF−ECF K balance or acid−base regulation. They are therefore included.

This book has been delayed in its completion but, as a result, it appears at a particularly important time. Until very recently few of the measurements which can really help to guide the choice of fluids and to monitor progress were readily available to general practice within a reasonable time, or at an acceptable cost. Now, however, plasma potassium is coming within reach of 'kit analysers' and above all, acid−base evaluation has become available in a rapid, precise, simple and inexpensive technique. An American humourist remarked, nearly 70 years ago, that 'life is a struggle not against sin, not against money power . . . but against hydrogen ions'. It is appropriate because being unable to measure conveniently acid−base balance, veterinary practice has scarcely taken it seriously. Yet whether we measure it or not, severe acidosis is lethal, e.g. in shock or in diarrhoea. 'The dying man doesn't struggle much and he isn't much afraid. As his alkalis give out he succumbs to a blest stupidity. His mind fogs. His will power vanishes. He submits decently. He scarcely gives a damn' (H.L. Mencken, 1919). At last we can stop apologizing for our inability to assess these crucial disturbances and allow our vital therapeutic choices to be guided by readily available measurements. More important, we can monitor progress, and as experience accumulates we will rapidly come to know which solutions work, and which do not.

Fluid therapy is not a panacea and it will not always succeed but, used appropriately, it ought to be effective, relatively inexpensive and almost without risk. We need to know about its shortcomings in order to improve its successes. We therefore hope that this book will not only encourage more veterinarians or prospective veterinarians to regard it as a subject which they understand and in which they trust their judgement rather than set recipes, but that it will also encourage practitioners to tell us about the problems which they encounter. Although a book of this length dealing with a variety of species must work through principles, rather than providing encyclopaedic detail, we would welcome suggestions for additional problems meriting discussion in any future editions.

There are three reasons why fluid therapy fails where it ought to succeed. The first is that insufficient or inappropriate fluids are given and the second that they are given too late or not persistently enough. These, the book can help to remedy. The third is that, as yet, we do not sufficiently understand the underlying pathophysiology; here too the book can help, but so can its readers by documenting their clinical experience.

A.R. MICHELL

Acknowledgements

We would like to acknowledge generous help and thank:
David Gunn (ABIPP), Tony Wagstaff, Portex, TMS Consultants and Murray Corke for providing illustrations;
Murray Corke for providing a detailed account of his approach to the preparation of sterile fluids;
Rosemary Forster for preparing the text and Rachel Nalumoso for sub-editing it.

The preparation of this book would have been very much harder without the magnificent library facilities and services of the Royal Society of Medicine.

Finally, we would like to acknowledge the particular impetus given to veterinary fluid therapy by John Watt, who was such a strong advocate of its potential in farm animals, in the early 1960s.

List of abbreviations

ACD	acid citrate dextrose
ADH	antidiuretic hormone
AMP	adenosine monophosphate
ARF	acute renal failure
BIC	bicarbonate (HCO_3^-)
BWt	body weight
CNS	central nervous system
CPD	citrate phosphate dextrose
CRT	capillary refill time
CSF	cerebrospinal fluid
CTZ	chemoreceptor trigger zone
CVP	central venous pressure
DEA	dog erythrocyte antigen
DIC	disseminated intravascular coagulation
DPG	diphosphoglycerate
ECF	extracellular fluid
ECG	electrocardiogram
EDTA	ethylenediaminetetra-acetic acid
ETEC	enterotoxigenic *Escherichia coli*
FFA	free fatty acid
FUS	feline urological syndrome
GFR	glomerular filtration rate
GMP	guanosine monophosphate
HES	hydroxyethylstarch
ICF	intracellular fluid
LDA	left displaced abomasum
LT	(heat) labile toxin
MDF	myocardial depressant factor
ORS	oral rehydration solution
Pao_2	partial pressure of arterial oxygen
Pco_2	partial pressure of carbon dioxide
Po_2	partial pressure of oxygen
PAWP	pulmonary artery wedge pressure
PCV	packed cell volume — haematocrit
PTH	parathyroid hormone
QRS	segment of electrocardiograph
RBC	red blood cells
RDA	right displaced abomasum
ST	(heat) stable toxin
TCO_2	total carbon dioxide (a measure of *metabolic* acidosis)
TP	total protein
TPN	total parenteral nutrition
WBC	white blood cells

Chapter 1
Regulation of body fluids

Introduction

Books on the kidney and regulation of body fluids tend to be long, detailed, and steeped in controversy. Yet the kidneys' role in regulating body fluids is reasonably clear — the uncertainties concern the details of how they actually operate [1]. It is over 150 years since Dr O'Shaughnessy, in a remarkable piece of clinical biochemistry, defined the main life-threatening consequences of dehydration induced by diarrhoea [2]; among them was clear evidence of functional renal failure. A decision to use fluid therapy implies that the renal mechanisms which defend body fluids are temporarily impaired or overwhelmed. The paramount objective of fluid therapy is not so much to treat the resulting abnormalities of plasma composition, unless they are extreme, but to restore the ability of the kidney to correct these disturbances. A healthy kidney — even one — can regulate the volume and composition of body fluids with a finesse envied by the finest fluid therapist supported by the most modern clinical laboratory. Indeed, once we humbly accept this point we become less dependent on the laboratory except to warn of dangerous extremes or confirm the effectiveness of therapy.

Most of what follows concerns the renal regulation of body fluids and thereby follows the conventional view of the subject. It is clear, however, that such preoccupation with the kidney has excessively diverted attention away from other aspects such as the importance of bone as a reservoir or a repository for excess salt, the importance of salt appetite in herbivores, or the importance of the gut, alongside the kidney in regulating body sodium and water [3−5]. No more will be said of this except to alert veterinarians to the well-kept secret that many animals, particularly herbivores, disregard the textbooks based on human physiology and excrete most of their sodium in faeces rather than urine, even when they are healthy [5].

1

Kidney and body fluids

The kidney is involved in the regulation of numerous aspects of plasma composition but those most relevant to the objectives of fluid therapy are the concentrations of sodium (Na), potassium (K) and hydrogen ions (H^+). The kidney is also important in regulating the concentration of divalent ions such as calcium (Ca) and magnesium (Mg), both of which are often the target of intravenous fluids although this is less often considered a part of fluid therapy. The key role of the kidney, however, is to regulate plasma volume because when this is ineffectively accomplished, or overwhelmed by disease, the animal confronts not only the threat of shock but also of a further decline in renal function, as a result of the reduction in circulating volume. Repair of circulating volume, 'volume replacement', is thus the key objective of fluid therapy, restoring to the kidney (and liver) the ability to regulate plasma composition. This explains the paradox that even solutions with slightly less sodium than normal plasma, can correct a fall in plasma sodium concentration. Furthermore, that correction of acidosis does not invariably require alkaline solutions, that alkalotic animals do not need acid, and that even animals with lactic acidosis may benefit from lactate-containing solutions [6–8].

In any fluid and electrolyte disturbance, it is essential to realize that the alterations in body fluids are not just the result of the pathological losses, e.g. the relative losses of salt and water in diarrhoeic faeces but also of the renal response which may be adaptive or, once overstretched, maladaptive. Thus animals which vomit lose relatively little potassium by this route yet they often become potassium depleted and hypokalaemic (low plasma K) as a result of their renal responses (see Chapter 2). Most animals with diarrhoea tend to become hyponatraemic (low plasma Na^+) rather than hypernatraemic yet their faeces rarely contain more salt than water and they certainly do not need hypertonic saline. The 'leaky radiator' approach to fluid therapy — top up with what was lost — is seldom correct. Living systems are more subtle and more robust.

Body water, Na and K

Water constitutes approximately 50–60% of the weight of an animal; more if it is young or lean, less if it is fat because fat contains no water. Although newborn animals may have considerably more than 70% or even 80% [9] of their weight as water, this proportion declines rapidly in the days following birth and then more steadily with growth. It never represents a significant additional 'protection' for the young, compared with the large deficits which they can incur, particularly with diarrhoea. Fluid losses amounting to 5% of normal body weight may be scarcely detectable, clinically, yet beyond 15% the animal is likely to be moribund, especially if the losses were rapid. Essentially, therefore, fluid therapy is concerned with deficits in the range 50−150 ml/kg body weight. An animal which loses fluids equivalent to 15% of body weight may have lost 25−30% of its body water — perhaps three times its plasma volume. The losses of a scouring animal may look less dramatic than a haemorrhage but no wonder they can be just as lethal.

Of the body water, most (66%) is inside cells — intracellular fluid (ICF). The extracellular fluid (ECF) is 20% of body weight, and most is in the tissue spaces (interstitial fluid) providing the environment of the cells and the transport system linking them with the blood vessels. Figure 1.1 shows the distribution of body water. The circulating portion of ECF, the plasma, is roughly 5−8% of body weight. Blood volume (roughly 10% of body weight) includes a portion of ICF (in the red cells) as well as plasma. These proportions serve as useful clinical generalizations despite some uncertainties, particularly differences between species, age groups, etc. The main uncertainties concern ECF; it is difficult to find an ECF marker which allows exact measurement of this compartment alone, particularly when permeabilities are altered by disease. In any case, some areas of ECF are relatively poorly accessible to 'markers' and are thus less rapidly, probably less importantly, involved in major clinical disturbances. ECF tends to expand during pregnancy but we do not know whether this is a necessary adaptation, or a reflection of excess salt intake. Since ICF is measured by subtracting ECF from total body water, it is affected by any errors in estimates of ECF.

Precise knowledge of these numbers is unimportant but a rough idea is essential; it does not matter whether the blood volume of a 4 kg cat is 400 ml or 450 ml nor whether that of a 400 kg horse is 39 l or 41 l; what matters is the order of magnitude. In particular, since no deficit below 5% body weight is likely to be clinically obvious, if we propose to give a litre of fluid to a carthorse we might as well apply it as a lotion since the minimum deficit worth treating would be around 25 l; in plasma alone the total likely deficit is 2−7 l.

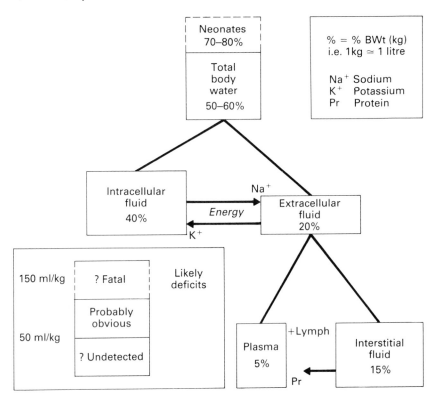

Fig. 1.1 Distribution of body water. For comparison: size of deficits.

The distribution of body water depends on osmotic gradients. Water crosses most cell membranes freely and moves rapidly to equalize the osmotic concentration between cells and their surroundings. By regulating the concentration of plasma, the kidney (and thirst) regulate the osmotic composition of both ECF and ICF. Disturbances of ECF osmotic composition, 'osmolality', cause cells to gain or lose water so regulation of ECF osmolality also stabilizes cell volume and abnormalities of ECF osmolality make cells swell or shrink. In most soft tissue the consequences may be mild but in brain, surrounded by a rigid cranium, they are potentially severe (Chapter 2).

Na and K

The main osmotic constituent of ICF is potassium; in ECF it is sodium and this balance is maintained by an energy-consuming enzyme system (Na−K ATPase; the 'sodium' pump) which not only extrudes sodium from cells but helps to bring in potassium. While consuming a major proportion of the available energy (ATP), this ubiquitous membrane pump creates gradients of Na and K which can then be used for the transfer of other solutes and of water, and, by moving more Na than K, establishes the voltages underlying the function of excitable tissues. It also prevents cells from swelling with excess water attracted by proteins and other solutes in ICF. When its functions fail or are undermined by membrane damage, plasma K rises, cells swell and plasma volume falls [10], *sick cell syndrome.*

Since intracellular volume is twice that of ECF and since ICF potassium concentration [K] is over 20 times that of normal plasma (Fig. 1.2), the distribution of K between ICF and ECF has a much more immediate impact on plasma K than that of renal excretion. Thus the treatment of hyperkalaemia aims to drive K back into cells or oppose its adverse effects; improved renal excretion is too slow (see Chapter 6). It only needs leakage of 2% of cell potassium to double plasma [K]. The sodium pump increases its activity directly with a rise in plasma K; insulin promotes this activity further and its secretion is increased during hyperkalaemia. β-adrenergic agonists also drive K^+ into cells. Aldosterone secretion from the adrenal cortex is directly stimulated by a rising plasma K. Thus there are several mechanisms contributing to the normal distribution of K; aldosterone also promotes K excretion, not only by increasing urinary losses but by moving K into gut fluids and skin secretions.

Sodium is kept largely in ECF by the Na pump and it is 'clothed' with the appropriate amount of water to maintain normal plasma [Na], and osmolality. Its concentration is thus regulated by the mechanisms controlling water intake and output, i.e. thirst and ADH (antidiuretic hormone). The immediate cause of an abnormal plasma [Na] is, therefore, abnormal water balance [11, 12]. Sodium acts as the osmotic skeleton of ECF, enabling it to hold its volume against the osmotic pull of the cell contents. Disturbances of body sodium primarily affect ECF volume and thereby plasma volume, hence their seriousness; effects on plasma sodium concentration, if any, are secondary [6, 12, 13].

Interstitial fluid

Stability of circulating volume depends on adequate ECF volume but the distribution between interstitial fluid (tissue fluid) and plasma is

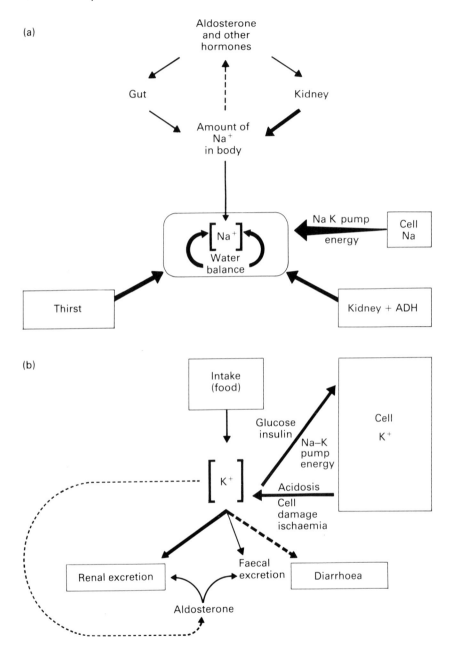

Fig. 1.2 Regulation of plasma: (a) Na^+ concentration; (b) K^+ concentration.

also crucial. Both are part of ECF so their main osmotic component is sodium. Plasma, however, contains more protein, notably albumin, than interstitial fluid and this provides an osmotic gradient which allows fluid to be retrieved into plasma at the venous end of the capillaries (Fig. 1.3). At the arterial end, the capillary hydrostatic pressure provides an outward force supplying fresh fluid to the interstitial compartment. There is thus a further circulatory system outside the blood vessels, supplying the cells. Not all this fluid is free, being adsorbed onto connective tissue components, and the diffusion distances between cells and capillaries are normally small. When excess free tissue fluid accumulates (oedema) exchange is thus impaired rather than improved. The presence of albumin in plasma also provides negative charges which hold additional Na^+, thus boosting its osmotic effect and reinforcing its role in supporting plasma volume.

The main factor preventing oedema is the protein osmotic gradient favouring uptake of fluid into capillaries. This depends on adequate concentration of plasma albumin and even more on low concentrations of interstitial protein. These low concentrations depend on the ability of the lymphatics to remove proteins 'spilled' from capillaries or cells

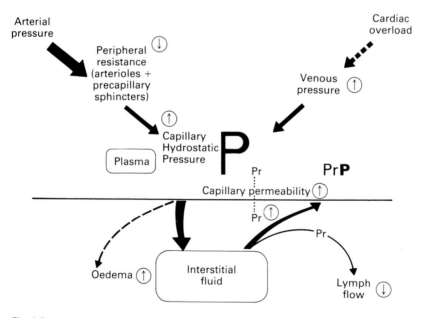

Fig. 1.3 Plasma, interstitial fluid and oedema. Factors affecting normal distribution: Pr = protein. Ringed arrows indicate factors contributing to oedema.

and to enhance their drainage if fluid starts to accumulate [14]. Thus lymphatic blockage or increased capillary permeability both cause oedema for the same reason; they raise the protein content of interstitial fluid. Peripheral oedema is cosmetic rather than life-threatening but it warns of an underlying abnormality. Pulmonary oedema, however, is life-threatening and can result from injudicious fluid therapy. This is considered further in Chapter 4 since shock, for various reasons, increases the possibility of pulmonary oedema. It is worth warning here, however, that the balance of the factors underlying pulmonary oedema is rather different from that in other tissues.

Units of measurement and factors affecting interpretation

Albumin is a more important protein, osmotically, than globulin because it is smaller. A given weight of albumin contributes more particles than globulin because each weighs less, and osmotic properties depend on the number of particles free in solution, regardless of their size or identity. For the same reason, sodium is far more effective as an osmotic constituent of plasma than albumin even though its concentration in g/l is much smaller. When capillaries are damaged albumin, rather than globulin, leaks into interstitial fluid because it is smaller.

The properties of solutions used in fluid therapy can only be understood when the composition is expressed in units reflecting the number of particles rather than the weight of each solute, i.e. mmol (millimole) rather than mg; it is therefore essential that manufacturers specify the composition *received by the animal* in mmol/l as well as any other information they give as mixing instructions [15].

For Na and K, chloride (Cl) and bicarbonate (BIC), the most important ions in fluid therapy, a mmol is the same as the molecular weight in mg; it is also the same as the now superseded mEq (milliequivalent). Since a mmol of sodium chloride yields a mmol of Na and a mmol of Cl, it yields 2 osmotically active mmol or mOsm (milliosmole). Thus since the formula weight (molecular weight) of NaCl is 58.5 (Na 23, Cl 35.5) 58.5 mg in 1 litre yields 1 mmol/l Na, 1 mmol/l Cl and 2 mOsm/l. A mmol of K is 39 mg, of bicarbonate 61 mg.

Depression of freezing point or elevation of boiling point also depend on the number of dissolved particles, regardless of type, hence they can be used in instruments to measure osmotic concentration directly, with a read-out in mOsm/l. The osmolality of a solution can also be calculated by converting all its major constituents from mg/l to mmol/l but this is laborious and less accurate because, for example, ECF is not dilute enough to allow salt to dissociate totally into free Na and Cl ions (though for practical purposes this can be ignored). Very approximately, the osmolality of plasma is double the sodium concentration. The term osmolality refers to a kg of solvent whereas the osmolarity is measured in a litre of solvent and therefore alters with temperature.

Divalent ions such as Ca and Mg can cause confusion. Firstly, one Ca ion will be associated with two Cl ions so 1 mmol of calcium chloride contains 1 mmol of Ca, 2 mmol of Cl and 3 mOsm of solute. Secondly, in the archaic units, 1 mmol of Ca represented 2 mEq. It is important to remember, both with Ca and Mg, that the freely ionized Ca or Mg is only part of the total. Much is bound to plasma proteins though this fraction does not affect (or cross) membranes. Hypocalcaemia, literally a fall in blood calcium, is clinically evident because of a fall in the freely ionized calcium which actually affects cells. Total calcium can alter simply because the albumin concentration alters but cells will remain unaffected unless free calcium also changes. Ion selective electrodes (ISEs) only 'see' the free, biologically active calcium and ignore the protein bound component. Na, K, Cl and BIC are not bound in plasma.

In most circumstances significant changes in osmolality reflect changes in the concentration of the main osmotic constituent of ECF which is Na. If glucose accumulates, however, it holds water (drawn from cells) and despite raising osmolality directly, it tends to dilute plasma Na. In fact if plasma Na were 'normal' despite a high glucose it suggests that without the hyperglycaemia, plasma Na would be increased. Although hyperglycaemia directly depresses plasma Na, glucose also holds extra water in urine and this osmotic diuresis tends to have the opposite effect on plasma Na, i.e. raises it. The effects of diabetes mellitus on plasma Na are, therefore, somewhat variable (see Chapter 12). Urea contributes to measured osmolarity but not to 'physiologically effective' osmolarity since, provided it accumulates gradually, it equalizes across cell membranes and does not, therefore, cause redistribution of water. The terms hypotonic and hypertonic refer to solutions which would cause water movement into or out of normal cells; an isotonic solution leaves cell water undisturbed because its osmotic concentration is identical to ICF. An isosmotic solution of urea, however, is not isotonic because it equilibrates between ECF and ICF and then exerts no osmotic effect — it is as if water alone had been added.

Even after removal of cells, plasma is not entirely aqueous; the proteins and lipids occupy a finite water-free space which is normally ignored. In severe hyperproteinaemia or hyperlipidaemia, the increase in this volume causes a fall in the aqueous volume. Since this contains the ions, analyses will show a fall in plasma sodium concentration which is spurious or 'factitious' because biological processes are only affected by the concentration in the aqueous phase which remains normal [16].

Acid–base balance

Just as plasma calcium is tied to albumin, hydrogen ions are tied to many chemical groups and it is only the minute concentration remaining free in plasma which establishes its pH, affects biological processes and registers with pH electrodes. Most of the hydrogen ions in plasma are tied to buffers allowing them to be carried from sites of generation to sites of excretion (kidney) without disturbing plasma pH. Similarly, urine transports large quantities of hydrogen ions tied to buffers; the amount excreted as *free* hydrogen ions, even at an 'acidic' pH of 4.5 is negligible — needing a gallon of unbuffered urine to excrete 0.5 ml of gastric acid [17].

In the presence of a weak (partially dissociated) acid, e.g. carbonic acid, the following equilibrium exists:

$$CO_2 + H_2O = H_2CO_3 \rightleftharpoons H^+ + HCO_3^- \tag{A}$$

Thus,

$$H^+ \propto \frac{H_2CO_3}{HCO_3^-} \tag{B}$$

i.e.

$$H^+ \propto \frac{PCO_2}{HCO_3^-} \tag{C}$$

Thus if the ratio of CO_2 and bicarbonate (BIC) is normal, pH is also normal even if PCO_2 and BIC, individually, are disturbed. The lungs and kidneys can directly alter CO_2 and BIC and thus influence H^+ (pH). This, rather than its chemical properties, makes the bicarbonate buffer system so important.

Acid–base balance is traditionally considered in terms of pH despite some advocates of mmol/l of H^+ [18]. Since pH is a negative log (log of reciprocal) of $[H^+]$, equation (C) is more usually presented thus:

$$pH = pK + \log \frac{[HCO_3]}{s \times P_{CO_2}} \tag{D}$$

where pK is a log of a dissociation constant and s is a solubility factor converting P_{CO_2} to mmol/l. This 'Henderson–Hasselbalch' equation, though more useful for calculation, is less helpful for understanding acid–base physiology; equation (C) is therefore used here for explanatory purposes.

Bicarbonate is the dominant buffer but haemoglobin is also important and behaves more like a conventional chemical buffer, taking up excess H^+ ions during acidosis and converting them into the harmless form HHb, no longer contributing to pH.

$$H^+ + Hb^- \rightleftharpoons HHb$$

If H^+ ions are scarce (alkalosis) HHb can dissociate to replace them. Haemoglobin is a special example of an intracellular buffer; there are many others including proteins and phosphates. Since ICF is much larger than ECF, the ability of excess H^+ to be buffered in ICF is an important part of the defense against acidosis; the price paid is that K moves out of cells as H^+ moves in, thus acidosis tends to cause hyperkalaemia even in animals with (cellular) K deficits (Chapter 2).

Renal function (Figure 1.4)

The kidneys continuously convert about 5% of cardiac output into protein-free primitive urine (glomerular filtrate). It is obviously vital that the majority is reabsorbed at a rate appropriate to the maintenance of normal plasma volume. This is accomplished in the proximal tubule which reabsorbs about 66% of the filtered Na and Cl, at unchanged concentration; reabsorption is enhanced by volume depletion and reduced by ECF volume expansion. The proximal tubule, therefore, readily defends plasma volume but not plasma composition which is much more dependent on processes 'downstream' in the nephron. It is thus possible for enhanced proximal reabsorption of Na, in defence of plasma volume, to undermine more distal reabsorptive processes

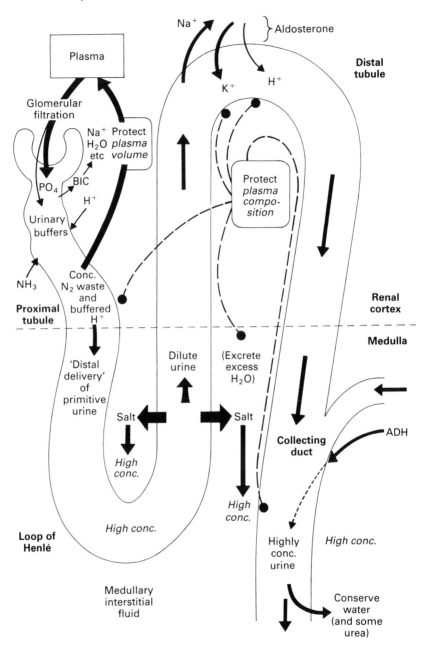

Fig. 1.4 Essentials of renal function in a single nephron.

which stabilize plasma composition [19, 20]; from the viewpoint of fluid therapy, this is probably the most important aspect of renal physiology [6]. During proximal reabsorption essential substances such as glucose and potassium are fully conserved, leaving nitrogenous waste such as urea and creatinine to become concentrated as urine volume falls. If glucose is delivered too fast, however, during hyperglycaemia, it appears in final urine. This explains not only the glycosuria of diabetes mellitus but also the constraints on the speed of glucose infusions, if they are to be effective.

The simple outcomes just described rest on a mass of unresolved controversies concerning underlying mechanisms which probably constitute the majority of research in renal physiology. We do not know how reabsorption is matched to filtration rate (or vice versa). We do not know how circulating volume is perceived — certainly by volume receptors on the venous side and baroreceptors on the arterial side including those in the renal arterioles. We do not know how important are the effects of renin/angiotensin generated in the kidney during poor perfusion, i.e. local effects, apart from promotion of aldosterone secretion or effects on systemic circulation. We know that the macula densa in the distal nephron senses the delivery of Na/Cl from the proximal tubule and loop of Henle but we remain uncertain how this information is used to stabilize perfusion, filtration, or reabsorption. We do not know how important are changes in the interstitial and capillary fluid composition around the tubules in resetting proximal reabsorption, e.g. increased capillary protein in providing a favourable reabsorptive gradient during volume depletion or increased filtration pressure (which could otherwise cause volume depletion). We do not know the importance of the substantial sympathetic innervation of renal tubules as well as vessels, though kidneys still function well when denervated (except during dehydration or anaesthesia). Nor is the role of prostaglandins clear, except perhaps in contributing to the ability of renal function to resist substantial falls in arterial pressure. What the kidney does is reasonably clear; fortunately, for the purposes of fluid therapy, we do not need to analyse the uncertainties surrounding the mechanisms involved [21−24].

Very recently some of the mechanisms enabling the kidney to excrete excess sodium have rapidly become clearer. Two types of 'natriuretic hormones' have been found, one originating from the brain and affecting sodium transport, the other from the atria of the heart and affecting glomerular filtration, sodium reabsorption and arterial pressure [1]. Their clinical importance is also emerging, in resisting sodium accumulation during congestive heart failure, chronic renal failure, and acute expansion of circulating volume, e.g. through excessive or over-rapid intravenous fluid therapy.

Loop: water conservation

In the loop of Henle, salt is extracted from the urine without water thus making the medullary interstitial fluid very concentrated (hypertonic) and the urine very dilute (hypotonic). If plasma becomes dilute the excess water can be excreted by leaving this hypotonic urine unmodified — except for some additional salt salvage in the distal nephron. If plasma becomes concentrated by water loss, urine needs to be concentrated in order to conserve water. This is accomplished by making the collecting ducts permeable; even in the cortex, interstitial fluid (at plasma concentration) is more concentrated than dilute urine so water is reabsorbed. But more powerful water conservation occurs in the medulla where the collecting ducts are surrounded by the concentrated interstitial fluid generated by the loops of Henle.

The factor that allows the ducts to become permeable and conserve water is ADH secreted from the posterior pituitary and responsive even to a 1% rise in osmolality. Like thirst, ADH primarily protects plasma osmolality but they are both stimulated by volume depletion, though less sensitively. In severe volume depletion, however, protection of plasma volume overrides protection of plasma osmolality, i.e. water is drunk and conserved even if plasma becomes diluted; this is the usual clinical cause of hyponatraemia.

Both glucocorticoids and calcium maintain partial impermeability of the collecting duct; excesses reduce permeability and cause polyuria (hence sufficient hypernatraemia to be corrected by polydipsia). Adrenal insufficiency, however, increases permeability and this contributes to the associated water retention (hyponatraemia). Normal renal water conservation also depends on the very low medullary perfusion which allows both interstitial fluid and plasma to remain concentrated by the action of the loops. Water retrieved from the collecting ducts is not trapped in interstitial fluid; it returns to plasma along the protein osmotic gradient as in other capillaries.

The actual details of medullary function are much more complicated [25, 26] and urea plays an important role in maintaining maximal concentrating function, being reabsorbed in parallel with water when ADH is active, and being present in medullary interstitial fluid at high concentrations [27]. Thus when final urine contains high concentrations of urea, as it should, it does not oppose water conservation since the surrounding interstitial fluid is also rich in urea.

When loop function is impaired, the kidney is neither able to dilute urine (excrete water) nor concentrate urine (conserve water) fully effectively. The polyuria of chronic renal failure results from a reduced population of intact loops to establish medullary hypertonicity (and from augmented filtration and flow rates in surviving nephrons). In volume depletion, loop function is impaired by reduced delivery of sodium from the proximal tubule (where reabsorption is increased) [28]. Thus even without increases in ADH, water is excreted less efficiently despite the hyponatraemia which results. Equally, if volume depletion is associated with hypernatraemia, renal water conservation is impaired because reduced sodium delivery from the proximal tubule restricts the effectiveness of loop function. In pyometra, endotoxaemia prevents a normal renal response to ADH (see Chapter 12). In Cushing's syndrome, excess glucocorticoid prevents the collecting duct from responding to ADH: in both cases, the outcome is polyuria (hence polydipsia).

Distal nephron: Na and K

Only a small proportion of sodium reabsorption occurs in the distal nephron (distal tubules + collecting ducts). Nevertheless this fraction is very important:

1 It enables daily urinary loss to be adjusted to balance daily intake, even allowing urine to be virtually free of sodium when intake is low or body sodium is depleted. This is regulated by aldosterone which is secreted faster when the adrenal cortex is stimulated by renin/ angiotensin which, in turn, is augmented by poorer renal perfusion during sodium depletion. Aldosterone also minimizes sodium loss in gut and skin secretions (Fig. 1.5).

2 Distal sodium reabsorption, under the influence of aldosterone, indirectly facilitates the excretion of K and H^+. Mild volume depletion thus causes potassium loss but severe volume depletion causes hyper-kalaemia by restricting sodium delivery to the distal nephron, by similarly impairing H^+ excretion and because the resulting acidosis tends to displace potassium from cells [29, 30]. A calf with severe

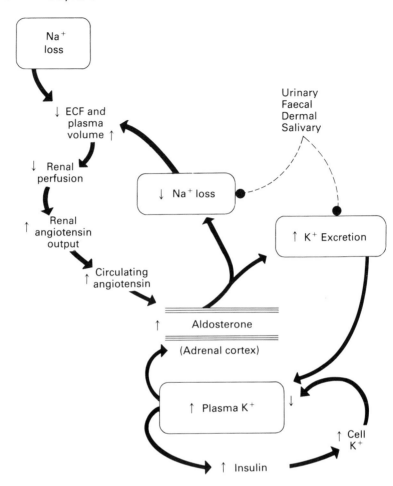

Fig. 1.5 ECF volume, aldosterone and plasma K$^+$.

diarrhoea may thus have hyperkalaemia despite its underlying deficit of cell K. Its ability to correct either hyperkalaemia or acidosis, renally, is restricted by the kidneys' response to volume depletion.

H$^+$ excretion (Figure 1.6)

Renal cells split carbonic acid to generate hydrogen ions for excretion and bicarbonate ions for the replenishment of plasma bicarbonate. Filtered bicarbonate is reabsorbed partly directly and partly by combining with some of the secreted H$^+$ to produce CO$_2$. This enters the

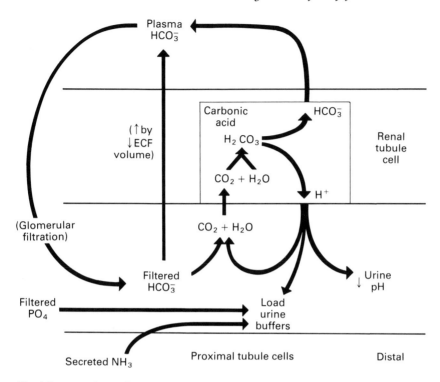

Fig. 1.6 Essentials of H⁺ excretion (and regulation of plasma bicarbonate).

tubular cell and provides more carbonic acid which, once split, provides a bicarbonate ion for reabsorption and a H⁺ which recycles into tubular fluid [31]. This process of bicarbonate reabsorption occurs in the proximal tubule and at a maximum rate which prevents plasma bicarbonate from rising above normal. The exception is during volume depletion. Thus even loss of acid, which tends to cause alkalosis, can be successfully countered by the kidney provided there is no volume depletion [32].

The other factor which can undermine the renal defence against alkalosis is potassium depletion [33]. Distal sodium reabsorption is enhanced by aldosterone and if K is depleted in renal cells, additional H⁺ is exchanged into urine instead of K. This 'paradoxical aciduria' (i.e. it worsens the alkalosis) is a typical feature of the metabolic alkalosis which frequently accompanies abomasal dysfunction in ruminants (see Chapter 12). If Cl is also depleted, as it is after vomiting, the alkalosis is aggravated because the negative ions accompanying reabsorbed Na will tend to be unwanted bicarbonate, rather than chloride. The correction of alkalosis is not, therefore, based on 'common sense' (replacement of acid) but on renal physiology (replacement of ECF volume, Cl and K, i.e. NaCl ± KCl).

Normal carnivore urine is acidic and the low pH is generated by H^+ secretion in the distal tubule. Proximal H^+ secretion helps bicarbonate reabsorption and also excretes large amounts of H^+ into urine but it is carried on the urinary buffers rather than free at low pH. These buffers are filtered phosphate and — traditionally — secreted ammonia (which generates ammonium ions in the tubule thus carrying H^+ in buffered form). Indeed aldosterone not only promotes distal secretion of H^+ but proximal generation of ammonia buffer (from glutamine) [34]. In ruminants the ammonia buffer, rather than phosphate, is important because substantial amounts of phosphate are secreted in saliva rather than appearing in urine [19]. Recently, however, these traditional views have been questioned, at least in carnivores, because a detailed consideration of the metabolic origin of the ammonia suggests that it generates as much H^+ as it transports [35]. Nevertheless, once present in urine, ammonia remains an important buffer.

Contraction of ECF volume tends to raise BIC concentration while $P\text{CO}_2$ remains stable; there is thus 'contraction alkalosis' and the kidney fails to lower the excess bicarbonate while volume depletion persists [36]. Equally well, however, if severe volume depletion is accompanied by bicarbonate loss and acidosis, the ability of the kidney to correct the acidosis is impaired by reduced sodium delivery to the distal nephron. Expansion of ECF volume with bicarbonate-free solutions, while improving renal function, will be less effective in correcting acidosis since the fluids will further dilute the remaining bicarbonate while the kidney strives to restore it. Indeed animals may end up rehydrated but still severely acidotic [37].

A number of anions such as lactate, citrate, acetate and propionate, once metabolized, leave equivalent amounts of bicarbonate and thus act as precursors. Lactate is particularly dependent on hepatic metabolism and underperfusion or liver disease may severely restrict its utilization. Healthy liver, properly perfused, however, has a massive capacity for metabolizing lactate and replacing it by bicarbonate [38]. Lactated solutions are therefore well utilized even by animals with lactic acidosis once perfusion recovers and provided liver function is intact. In fact it is increasingly being realized that the liver, alongside the kidney, has an important role in acid–base regulation. This arises particularly from the fact that hepatic conversion of ammonia to urea consumes bicarbonate, whereas conversion to glutamine does not [39].

Conclusion

The ability of the proximal tubule to defend against volume depletion is based on enhanced sodium reabsorption. This reduces the effectiveness, however, of the defence of plasma composition by subsequent segments of the nephron. Such *sequential imbalance* of renal function impairs the regulation of plasma Na, K, Cl, H^+ and BIC, i.e. the ions which are the main concern of fluid therapy. Moreover in veterinary practice the ability to obtain laboratory data about these ions is often restricted. The repair of extracellular volume depletion is therefore the cardinal priority of fluid therapy, helping the kidney itself to restore plasma composition.

References

1 Michell, A.R. (1988) Renal function, renal damage and renal failure. In: *Renal Disease in Dogs and Cats*, 5–29. Michell, A.R. (ed). Blackwell Scientific Publications, Oxford.

2 O'Shaughnessy, W.B. (1832) *Report on the Chemical Pathology of Malignant Cholera*. S. Highley, London.

3 Michell, A.R. (1976) Skeletal sodium, a missing element in hypertension and salt excretion. *Perspectives in Biology and Medicine* **20**, 27–33.

4 Michell, A.R. (1978) Salt appetite, sodium metabolism and hypertension: a deviation of perspective. *Perspectives in Biology and Medicine* **21**, 335–47.

5 Michell, A.R. (1985) The gut, the unobtrusive regulator of sodium balance. *Perspectives in Biology and Medicine* **29**, 203–13.

6 Michell, A.R. (1979) The pathophysiological basis of fluid therapy in small animals. *Veterinary Record* **104**, 542–8.

7 Michell, A.R. (1985) What is shock? *Journal of Small Animal Practice* **26**, 719–38.

8 Michell, A.R. (1988) Drips, drinks and drenches; what matters in fluid therapy? *Irish Veterinary Journal* **42**, 17–22.

9 Thornton, J.R. & English, P.B. (1978) Body water of calves; changes in distribution with diarrhoea. *British Veterinary Journal* **134**, 445–53.

10 Flear, C.T.G. (1970) Electrolyte and body water changes after trauma. *Journal of Clinical Pathology* (Suppl.) **4**, 16–31.

11 Shapiro, J.I. & Anderson, R.J. (1987) In: *Body Fluid Homeostasis*, 245–76. Brenner, B.M. & Stein, J.H. (eds). Churchill Livingstone, New York.

12 Gardenswartz, M.H. & Schrier, R.W. (1982) In: *Sodium, its Biological Significance*, 19–74. Papper, S. (ed.). C.R.C., Florida.

13 Greenberg, A. (1985) In: *Disorders of Fluid and Electrolyte Balance*, 137–60. Puschett, J.B. (ed.). Churchill Livingstone, New York.

14 Guyton, A.C. (1986) *Textbook of Medical Physiology*, 361–70. W.B. Saunders, Philadelphia.

15 Michell, A.R. (1983) Understanding fluid therapy. *Irish Veterinary Journal* **37**, 94−103.

16 Walmsley, R.N. & Guerin, M.D. (1984) *Disorders of Fluid and Electrolyte Balance*, 36. Wright, Bristol.

17 Michell, A.R. (1980) The kidney: regulation and disturbances of body fluids. In: *Physiological Basis of Small Animal Medicine*, 71−126. Yoxall, A.T. & Hird, J.F.R. (eds). Blackwell Scientific Publications, Oxford.

18 Michell, A.R. (1970) Protons, pH and survival. *Journal of the American Veterinary Medicine Association* **157**, 1540−8.

19 Michell, A.R. (1983) In: *Veterinary Nephrology*, 57−71. Hall, L.W. (ed). Heinemann, London.

20 Vaamonde, C.A. (1982) In: *Sodium, its Biological Significance*, 208−37. Papper, S. (ed). C.R.C. Press, Florida.

21 Raymond, K.H. & Stein, S.H. (1987) In: *Body Fluid Homeostasis*, 33−68. Brenner, B.M. & Stein, J.H. (eds). Churchill Livingstone, New York.

22 Kopp, V.C. & Di Bona, G.F. (1987) In: *Body Fluid Homeostasis*, 185−220. Brenner, B.M. & Stein, J.H. (eds). Churchill Livingstone, New York.

23 Schlondorff, D. & Ardaillou, R. (1986) Prostaglandin and other arachidonic acid metabolites in the kidney. *Kidney International* **29**, 108−19.

24 Marsden, P.A. & Skorecki, K.L. (1987) In: *Body Fluid Homeostasis*, 1−32. Brenner, B.M. & Stein, J.H. (eds). Churchill Livingstone, New York.

25 De Rouffignac, C. & Jamison, R.L. (1987) The urinary concentrating mechanism. *Kidney International* **31**, 501−672.

26 Bankir, L., Bouby, N., Tan, M.T. & Kaissling, B. (1987) The thick ascending limb. *Advances in Nephrology* **16**, 69−102.

27 Knepper, M.A. & Roch-Ramel, F. (1987) Pathways of urea transport in the mammalian kidney. *Kidney International* **31**, 629−33.

28 Greenberg, A. (1985) In: *Disorders of Fluid and Electrolyte Balance*, 113−36. Puschett, J.B. (ed). Churchill Livingstone, New York.

29 Kaufman, C.E. & Papper, S. (1983) In: *Potassium: its Biological Significance*, 77−92, Whang, R.D. (ed). C.R.C. Press, Florida.

30 Cox, M. (1981) Potassium homeostasis. *Medical Clinics of North America*, **65**, 363−84.

31 O'Connor, G. & Kunau, R.T. (1978) In: *Acid−Base and Potassium Homeostasis*, 1−29. Brenner, B.M. & Stein, J.H. (eds). Churchill Livingstone, New York.

32 Carroll, H.J. & Oh, M.S. (1978) *Water, Electrolyte and Acid−Base Metabolism*, 261−77. Lippincott, Philadelphia.

33 Dubose, T.D. (1981) Metabolic alkalosis. *Seminars in Nephrology* **1**, 281−9.

34 Batlle, D.C. (1981) Hyperkalemic hyperchloraemic metabolic acidosis with aldosterone deficiency. *Seminars in Nephrology* **1**, 260−74.

35 Halperin, M.L. & Jungas, R.L. (1984) Metabolic production and renal disposal of hydrogen ions. *Kidney International* **24**, 709−13.

36 Cohen, J.J. & Kassirer, J.P. (1982) *Acid Base*, 121−6. Little Brown & Co, Boston.

37 Kasari, T.R. & Naylor, J.M. (1986) Further studies of a syndrome of metabolic acidosis with minimal dehydration in neonatal calves. *Canadian Journal of Veterinary Research* **50**, 502−8.

38 Brautbar, N. (1981) Extrarenal factors in the homeostasis of acid−base balance. *Seminars in Nephrology* **1**, 232−49.

39 Atkinson, D.E. & Camien, M.N. (1982) The role of urea synthesis in the removal of metabolic bicarbonate and the regulation of blood pH. *Current Topics in Cellular Regulation* **21**, 261−301.

Chapter 2
Disturbances of volume and composition of body fluids

Introduction

Most disturbances of extracellular fluid volume are accompanied by disturbances of plasma composition. As already explained, this is not only because of ionic losses contributing to the initial problem but because the renal defence against volume depletion impairs the kidney's ability to regulate plasma composition. Restoration of ECF volume with plasma-like solutions can therefore bring about disproportionate improvements in plasma composition and, for example, neutral solutions can improve both alkalosis and acidosis. Similarly, a fall in plasma sodium concentration does not demand that solutions with elevated sodium content are required for therapy.

This chapter briefly surveys the 'pure' disturbances of volume and composition which form the specific targets for fluid therapy. It then considers the combined disturbances which are characteristically caused by some major groups of clinical conditions. Finally, it illustrates how the appropriate fluid therapy for any clinical requirement can be reasonably assessed from a consideration of the likely combination of disturbances. The emphasis is mainly, though not exclusively, on this approach rather than the use of laboratory data since their availability is usually restricted or slow in veterinary practice. Wherever possible, it is important that opportunities are taken to use laboratory data to confirm the assumptions based on history and clinical presentation, as well as the degree of improvement achieved by treatment. Such use of the laboratory where available will ultimately allow greater confidence in predictions and decisions made without it. Successful fluid therapy with or without the laboratory rests above all on adequate repair of extracellular volume and the fact that it allows the healthy kidney to resume the normal regulation of plasma composition.

Where there is underlying renal disease the ability to compensate either for disease or misguided fluid therapy is reduced. Unfortunately, because the kidney compensates so successfully for its own progressive loss of function in chronic renal failure [1], the existence of renal disease is not clinically obvious until it is well advanced, or revealed by a restricted ability to cope with dehydration or fluid overload (see Chapter 10). Nevertheless, it is important to realize that dehydration can also cause sufficient impairment of renal function, even in healthy kidneys, to allow a rise in plasma urea concentration — as observed in 1831 by O'Shaughnessy in his classical study of the effects of cholera diarrhoea [2]. As we now know, this reflects not only reduced renal perfusion but the fact that the reabsorption of water and urea both increase in parallel during dehydration (see Chapter 1).

Volume depletion: plasma sodium: water loss

Since sodium is the osmotic skeleton of ECF (Chapter 1) the severity of volume depletion generally reflects the underlying loss of sodium. If there is pure water loss, the impact will be shared by all compartments in proportion to their size (Fig. 2.1). Thus, at 5% loss of body weight in a 50 kg animal, the total deficit is 2.5 l; 1.7 l (66%) from ICF, 0.8 l from ECF and of this only 0.2 l (25% of ECF) from plasma. If we assume that blood volume is roughly 10% of body weight, it becomes obvious that a loss of 0.2 l from an initial circulating volume of about 5 l will scarcely be devastating.

The clinical term 'dehydration' is not restricted to water deficits. Indeed, pure dehydration in this literal sense is probably less usual, though it is no less important. It occurs in conditions such as fever, chronic renal failure, heat stress, water deprivation, i.e. whenever drinking cannot keep pace with normal or abnormal losses (see Chapter 6). Although renal and faecal water losses are regulated (in the absence of renal or enteric disease) dermal and respiratory losses are not. Since urinary and faecal losses are seldom zero, simple water deprivation can easily reduce body water by more than 25 ml/kg/day. Any condition which interferes with the release of ADH or the ability of the kidney to produce concentrated urine can greatly increase these losses, e.g. K^+ depletion, hypercalcaemia, pyometra, inadequate protein intake (by reducing urea production), Cushing's syndrome. Increased respiratory loss of water can also be important, especially at high temperatures and low humidity. Even in the absence of sweating, dermal losses can be substantial, especially with extensive wounds. Thus, cessation of drinking or inadequate drinking (pain, weakness) can rapidly produce clinically important water deficits without any

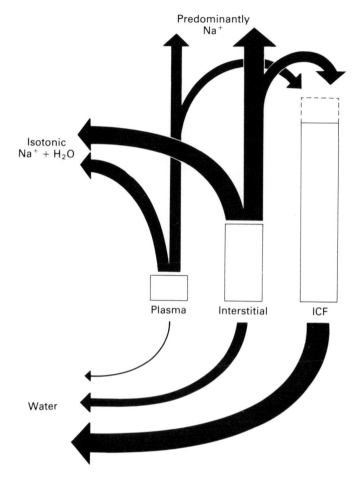

Fig. 2.1 Source of deficit: water and salt loss.

obvious source of abnormal loss, and information about fluid intake is a crucial part of the case history. The hallmark of pure water depletion is an elevated plasma sodium concentration (though it can also arise from ingestion or administration of excess salt).

Most clinical conditions, however, involve an accompanying loss of electrolytes, notably sodium. If the total sodium deficit accompanying water loss were isotonic (i.e. the same concentration as plasma) plasma sodium concentration would be unchanged but for precisely this reason the entire deficit would be borne by ECF. The cells (ICF) yield no water when the concentration of their surroundings is unchanged. The 2.8 l therefore comes entirely from ECF, 0.7 l from plasma, i.e. for the same change in body weight the impact on plasma is over three times as severe.

If there is a predominant loss of salt (i.e. plasma sodium concentration falls) the situation is far worse. ECF is then not only depleted by the external losses but by its inability to hold water against the osmotic pull of the ICF. Water enters cells (Fig. 2.1) until the osmotic concentration of both ICF and ECF is equal (both reduced). A low plasma sodium concentration, therefore, tells us that osmotic concentration is low throughout the body fluids and that intracellular fluid has increased its volume at the expense of ECF. Indeed, cells will swell, including brain cells in the rigid cranium and also red blood cells (RBC) which will therefore exaggerate the increased packed cell volume (PCV) by adding cell swelling to diminished plasma volume.

Depletion of ECF volume can also be exaggerated by loss of fluid into cells when they fail to eject sodium efficiently and allow it to increase in ICF. This can occur in underperfused tissue with inadequate delivery of substrates and oxygen leading to depressed sodium pump activity, e.g. in shock [3]. It may also be caused by increased permeability of cell membranes following ischaemia [4].

In external haemorrhage or diarrhoea fluid loss is clearly occurring but none is apparent with alimentary obstruction, extensive contusions or closed fractures. Areas of severe tissue damage allow substantial accumulations of additional interstitial fluid (including inflammatory exudates) and although this fluid is still within the body (and the ECF) it is no longer available to the circulation from which it originated. There is thus depletion of plasma volume which, if severe, will cause shock. Similarly, obstructed gut accumulates fluid and gas and can rapidly deplete plasma volume.

Sometimes there is increased defence of plasma volume without any readily detectable change in plasma volume. In oedema (or ascites), for example, the expansion of interstitial fluid at the expense of plasma can only continue because plasma volume is repleted by the kidney, i.e. the kidney is always the 'enabling' cause of oedema [5]. It can also be the primary cause (extensive protein leakage in glomerulonephritis, occasionally excess salt retention). The continuing depletion and repletion of plasma volume may sufficiently enhance thirst and ADH to depress plasma sodium concentration. Water retention in defence of subtle changes of plasma volume is also thought to underlie the fall of plasma sodium concentration which can accompany cardiac and hepatic failure [6–8]. In this case it is believed that total plasma volume may actually be normal but 'effective' plasma volume is reduced by depressed cardiac output or localized intravascular pooling. The defence of plasma volume is therefore activated.

The threat to plasma volume is always most severe when there is loss of plasma protein (albumin) since this provides the osmotic gradient for retrieving fluid from the tissue spaces (Chapter 1). Liver disease (impaired synthesis) therefore makes animals more susceptible to volume depletion. Extensive burns, though less usual in animals than humans, cause severe hypovolaemia by allowing leakage of protein-rich fluid from damaged capillaries.

Hyponatraemia and hypernatraemia

So far hyponatraemia has been considered almost entirely in the context of volume depletion which is by far its commonest cause (Fig. 2.2). It has been emphasized that it is caused not so much by pathological losses containing more sodium than plasma (which would make it unusual) but by water retention in defence of plasma volume (thirst and ADH). It could be caused by over-hydration [9] but since this would need to interfere with both thirst and ADH to cause significant water retention, the most likely cause would be excess fluid therapy [10]. The combination of stress, visceral traction and anaesthesia can, for example, provide 'irrelevant' stimuli for ADH secretion during and after surgery, apart from any real dehydration; excessive use of sodium-free fluids will then carry a risk of hyponatraemia [11] (see Chapter 11).

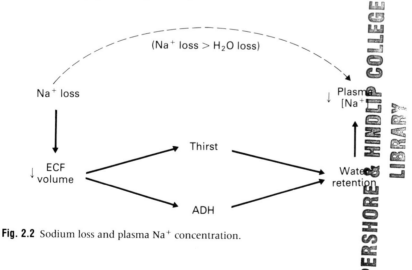

Fig. 2.2 Sodium loss and plasma Na$^+$ concentration.

Severe hyponatraemia (below 130 mmol/l) can cause a wide range of non-specific clinical symptoms including disturbances of intestinal and neurological function [12, 13]. This will require expansion of ECF with sodium-rich fluids (e.g. 'normal' saline with additional bicarbonate; Chapter 3). In the unusual instance that the problem is truly dilutional rather than a result of dehydration, there needs to be sufficient restriction of oral fluids to cause a slight daily loss of body weight (1−2%) [9]. Not only is this unusual but very difficult to manage without frequent measurement of plasma electrolyte concentration. Moreover, hyponatraemic dogs may be more susceptible to the effects of dehydration, with poorer urinary concentrating capacity [14]. Since the fundamental cause of hyponatraemia is usually hypovolaemia and rarely overhydration, there is almost no indication for the use of strongly hypertonic saline solutions in its treatment.

Severe hypernatraemia (above 160 mmol/l) can also cause a wide range of non-specific clinical symptoms including the characteristic convulsions of salt poisoning, e.g. in pigs and calves [12, 15, 16]. Partly these arise from cell shrinkage. During sustained hypernatraemia brain cells adapt by generating additional organic solutes [12], 'idiogenic osmoles', so that rapid rehydration (e.g. sudden drinking) will then allow excessive intracellular water uptake and precipitate severe neurological disturbances. Whenever hypernatraemia is detected the fundamental question is 'What prevented its correction by thirst?' Even the severe water losses of diabetes insipidus can usually be corrected by thirst without causing hypernatraemia.

Potassium

Unlike sodium, which is essentially an extracellular ion, potassium is predominantly intracellular but its plasma concentration must remain neither too high nor too low. Cell potassium mainly reflects the balance between intake and excretory or other losses; potassium depletion can produce substantial cell deficits but will not necessarily reduce plasma K. Even during potassium depletion, acidosis can drive sufficient hydrogen ions into cells and cause hyperkalaemia by displacement of K into plasma. Similarly, underperfused tissues leak K either because their Na−K pumps lack ATP or because hypoxia, like any other cause of cell damage, allows membranes to leak potassium (see Chapter 1).

The main causes of potassium deficits are anorexia, mild volume depletion (by increasing urinary excretion; Chapter 1) and additional losses in diarrhoeic faeces. The greater the underlying cell deficits, the greater the likelihood that there is also hypokalaemia. In particular, improvement of perfusion and correction of acidosis can rapidly convert hyperkalaemia to hypokalaemia in animals with potassium depletion [5, 17] Diuretics can also cause K deficits by inducing volume depletion [15]. The clinical effects of potassium depletion and hypokalaemia are numerous and varied but not diagnostically distinctive with the exception of ECG changes. Muscle weakness, both skeletal and smooth, is prominent, together with cardiac dysrhythmias and impairment of renal water conservation [18−20].

The main causes of potassium retention are severe volume depletion (by reducing the delivery of sodium to the distal nephron; Chapter 1) and acute renal failure (Chapter 10). An additional cause of hyperkalaemia is leakage of K from RBC either in the animal (intravascular haemolysis) or in sampling as a result of cell damage or cooling. This does not apply to dogs, cattle or most sheep whose RBC are unusual in having a low K content except when immature. Measurement of RBC K^+ has been exploited to assess the severity of K depletion in horses [21] (Chapter 5) which do have high K RBC.

Since aldosterone is a major regulator of sodium retention and potassium excretion (Chapter 1) adrenal insufficiency causes severe hypovolaemia and hyperkalaemia whereas excess secretion causes hypokalaemia and potassium depletion. Diabetes mellitus causes hyperkalaemia both through acidosis and the reduced levels of insulin available to promote cellular uptake of potassium (see Chapter 12).

Classification of acid−base disturbances

Plasma pH is normal, provided the ratio of P_{CO_2} and bicarbonate (HCO_3) is normal (Chapter 1). Disturbances of acid−base balance are therefore described as respiratory (if they arise from an abnormal P_{CO_2}) or metabolic (if they arise from abnormal HCO_3). A respiratory disturbance can be compensated by a parallel renal adjustment of plasma bicarbonate and similarly a metabolic disturbance can be compensated by a parallel adjustment of P_{CO_2}, thus returning the ratio (and hence pH) towards normal. Compensation is usually incomplete but serves to minimize the disturbance of pH. The four primary acid−base disorders (Fig. 2.3) are:

1 Metabolic acidosis implies a *primary loss or consumption of bicar-*

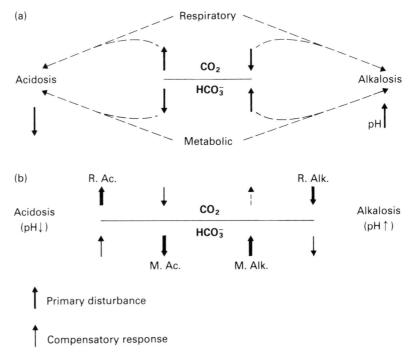

Fig. 2.3 (a) Primary acid−base disturbances; (b) compensatory responses.

bonate (by acid) and *pH usually falls* despite a prompt increase in pulmonary ventilation which produces the compensatory fall in P_{CO_2}.

2 Metabolic alkalosis implies a *primary excess of bicarbonate* (usually resulting from loss or pooling of gastric acid). *Almost invariably* pH rises because the compensatory response (depressed ventilation to raise P_{CO_2}) is restricted by the demands for adequate oxygenation.

3 Respiratory alkalosis implies a *fall in* P_{CO_2} due to hyperventilation (contrast metabolic alkalosis); there is renal compensation, i.e. a reduced plasma bicarbonate (contrast metabolic alkalosis).

4 Respiratory acidosis implies defective pulmonary ventilation or gas exchange leading to *increased* P_{CO_2} (contrast metabolic acidosis). The renal response is bicarbonate retention (contrast metabolic acidosis).

Since the respiratory conditions are not normally treated by fluid therapy they are not considered further except that they may complicate metabolic disturbances. Thus, they may reinforce a metabolic disturbance or prevent it from undergoing compensation. Anaesthesia, pulmonary disease or impaired pulmonary ventilation may therefore intensify the effects of metabolic disturbances and restrict the ability of the animal to resist incorrect fluid therapy.

Two acid—base disturbances may occur simultaneously and cancel out. Thus, with diarrhoea and vomiting there is loss of both alkali and acid or with gastric torsion there is sequestration of acid in the dilated stomach but generation of acid in ischaemic tissues as a result of shock. A respiratory alkalosis resulting from hyperventilation, e.g. during fever, could cancel out a metabolic acidosis caused by diarrhoea. On the other hand, a respiratory acidosis due to severe pneumonia could cancel out any alkalosis due to vomiting. (Pneumonia can cause respiratory alkalosis rather than acidosis, depending whether the predominant effect is to cause hyperventilation or impaired gas exchange; CO_2 diffuses more readily than O_2.)

Since pH is proportional to the ratio of $HCO_3 : Pco_2$ the assessment of acid—base status requires a measurement of two out of these three variables (see Chapter 5). At normal pH, however, the ratio is about $20 : 1$, once Pco_2 is converted to mmol/l, i.e. it is heavily dominated by bicarbonate. If we are mainly interested in metabolic disturbances rather than respiratory (Pco_2) changes, a measure of bicarbonate alone is useful and simple to perform (Chapter 5). Although called 'total CO_2' such a measure is obtained by strong acidification which converts bicarbonate to CO_2 and also liberates the original CO_2. The latter is only a minor contribution so the volume of CO_2 obtained essentially provides a measure of bicarbonate.

Metabolic acidosis

Is the most important acid—base disturbance requiring fluid therapy. By definition, plasma bicarbonate is reduced:
1 Because hydrogen ions have accumulated.
2 Because bicarbonate has been lost.
3 Because bicarbonate has been diluted.

H^+ accumulation

Hydrogen ions accumulate during renal failure but only slowly; if H^+ generation is about 1 mmol/kg/day and extracellular bicarbonate is about 5 mmol/kg, it would take several days of total cessation of renal H^+ excretion to produce severe acidosis [22]. On the other hand in chronic renal failure there is also chronic metabolic acidosis leading to bone damage, inappetance and other adverse effects (see Chapter 10). Quite apart from any specific defects in acidification of urine, the reduction in healthy renal tissue diminishes the supply of urinary buffers which arise from glomerular filtration (phosphate) and tubular synthesis (ammonia) [23, 24].

Since oxidative metabolism inescapably generates H^+ [25, 26], any acceleration of catabolism increases the endogenous generation of acid, especially if there is a resulting accumulation of organic acids [27]. This occurs with the production of acetoacetate and hydroxybutyrate during ketosis associated with starvation, diabetes mellitus, bovine acetonaemia and ovine pregnancy toxaemia.

Tissue hypoxia also causes acidosis by increasing the generation of lactic acid and its effects are intensified by hepatic disease or impaired hepatic perfusion since the liver can normally metabolize large quantities of lactate [28] (Chapter 1). Shock is therefore a powerful cause of metabolic acidosis (Chapter 4) although occasionally it can result in respiratory alkalosis because of hyperventilation [29]. Another cause of lactic acidosis is fermentation of excess grain in ruminants (see Chapter 12).

Bicarbonate loss

The main cause of bicarbonate loss is diarrhoea; intestinal obstruction can cause accumulation of bicarbonate within the obstructed gut but ischaemia and lactic acid production cause additional accumulation of hydrogen ions. Genetic defects or toxic damage to the proximal tubules can impair renal bicarbonate reabsorption and thus cause 'renal' acidosis [30]. Diuretics which inhibit carbonic anhydrase (e.g. acetazolamide) will also cause urinary bicarbonate wasting.

Since sodium reabsorption can be accompanied by either bicarbonate or chloride, disturbance of one of these anions tends to cause a reciprocal change in the plasma concentration of the other. Thus bicarbonate loss tends to cause a rise in plasma chloride concentration, and the other (unmeasured) anions are unaffected (Fig. 2.4). On the other hand, when the cause of metabolic acidosis is accumulation of hydrogen ions, there will also be an accumulation of the anions of the equivalent acids. The fall in plasma bicarbonate thus leads to a reciprocal rise in chloride when metabolic acidosis is caused by loss of bicarbonate but to a reciprocal rise in (unmeasured) anions when the

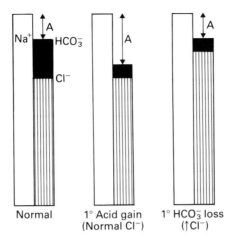

Fig. 2.4 Metabolic acidosis and anion gap.

cause is accumulation of acid [31]. This allows the cause of a metabolic acidosis to be interpreted from the laboratory measurement of 'anion gap' (Chapter 5) as well as clinical history.

Dilution

Administration of excess bicarbonate-free fluids, by diluting ECF bicarbonate, leads to metabolic acidosis because CO_2, being regulated by the respiratory centres, is not diluted. Nevertheless, in a dehydrated animal, bicarbonate-free fluids may improve plasma pH despite their composition, by improving renal perfusion. Sometimes clinicians are concerned to discover that an i.v. fluid may, for example, have a pH of 4. Since this represents 0.1 mmol of H^+/l, it would take 400 l to cause significant acidosis (reduce bicarbonate by 10 mmol/l) in a 20 kg animal; dilution, in fact drowning would be the problem, long before the pH.

Effects of acidosis

The persistence of metabolic acidosis has numerous adverse effects which are listed in Table 2.1. They are included not just for interest but also to emphasize that it is an important and life-threatening condition, regardless of the initiating cause. The fact that practical problems have deterred veterinary practitioners from assessing acid–base

Table 2.1 Some potential adverse effects of acidosis

1	Reduced oxygen uptake by haemoglobin
2	Initial respiratory stimulation then deep, slow gasping
3	Depression of vasomotor centre
4	Depression of myocardium
5	Increased red cell rigidity
6	Venoconstriction (impedes i.v. fluid administration)
7	Interferes with clotting
8	Exacerbates hyperkalaemia
9	Affects distribution of drugs (e.g. barbiturates) and action of hormones
10	Depresses glycolysis, alters enzyme activity, affects shape and charge of proteins
11	If sustained, bone damage

disturbances does not make them any less important; hydrogen ions become lethal whether or not we measure their concentration. Like disturbances of plasma Na^+ and K^+, acid−base disturbances produce a wide range of clinical signs and these are discussed in Chapter 5. Unfortunately, few are diagnostic and acid−base evaluation rests on clinical history and laboratory measurements. Among these, simple, rapid, accurate measurement of total CO_2 (Chapter 5) has the potential to revolutionize the management of acid−base disturbances in every-day veterinary practice [32].

Correction of acidosis

An established metabolic acidosis does not only affect the composition of plasma; cerebrospinal fluid undergoes parallel changes in CO_2 (rapidly) and bicarbonate (more gradually). A similar delay occurs in response to therapy, i.e. instantaneous restoration of normal P_{CO_2} and bicarbonate in plasma would leave CSF with normal CO_2 but still with depleted bicarbonate. The CSF would therefore remain acidic and maintain a now unwanted hyperventilation [33]. Metabolic acidosis must therefore be corrected more gradually to allow CSF bicarbonate to keep pace with the recovery in P_{CO_2} (which itself represents the dwindling respiratory compensation as the acidosis subsides). This, as well as the more obvious risk of miscalculation and overdose, provides an important reason for initially aiming at partial rather than total correction of metabolic acidosis [34]. Provision of bicarbonate as a precursor (lactate, acetate, etc.; Chapters 1 and 6) minimizes these risks [35].

Metabolic alkalosis

Whatever causes metabolic alkalosis, it is sustained by the renal effects of contraction in ECF volume, otherwise the kidney can readily resist rises in plasma bicarbonate [36]. The usual cause is that acid is sequestered in an obstructed and dilated stomach (or abomasum), or it is lost by vomiting. In both cases the accompanying volume depletion sustains the alkalosis and the fact that chloride is in short supply makes matters worse by encouraging retention of even more bicarbonate.

Generally, renal cells will undergo reciprocal changes in K^+ and H^+ thus making it easier for potassium to be available for urinary excretion during alkalosis, and metabolic alkalosis therefore tends to cause potassium depletion. It seems equally obvious that potassium depletion, by allowing more hydrogen ions to enter urine, will facilitate the development of alkalosis and thus complete the vicious cycle. Certainly such a 'paradoxical' aciduria can occur during metabolic alkalosis. Nevertheless, more recent observations indicate that potassium depletion need not invariably cause alkalosis, indeed in dogs the chronic effect may rather be to cause acidosis [37, 38]. It remains true, however, that metabolic alkalosis and potassium depletion frequently coexist because the former causes the latter.

Compensation

There are physiological constraints on the compensatory responses to metabolic alkalosis. Ventilation is depressed and $P\mathrm{co}_2$ rises, as required, but this will ultimately be over-ruled by the adverse effect on oxygenation; this is particularly important because alkalosis also impedes the release of oxygen from haemoglobin. Increased $P\mathrm{co}_2$ helps the kidney to retain bicarbonate, which is part of the compensatory response to respiratory acidosis but another limitation on the response to metabolic alkalosis, since additional bicarbonate reinforces the disturbance.

Correction

Since the kidney normally regulates bicarbonate effectively, the repair of metabolic alkalosis does not demand replacement of acid but rather the correction of the factors impeding renal regulation. These are mainly volume depletion and chloride depletion, possibly potassium depletion. Saline, with or without K^+, is thus appropriate despite being chemically neutral.

COMPOUND DISTURBANCES; CLINICAL SYNDROMES

The 'pure' disturbances underlying the clinical indications for fluid therapy have been described (except for those relating to nutrition, i.e. parenteral provision of calories, nitrogen, etc.; Chapter 12). In reality, they seldom arise in isolation and particular combinations are characteristically associated with various clinical syndromes. Some are described in brief, together with the appropriate therapy in Chapters 9 and 12. Those associated with anaesthesia and surgery are discussed in Chapter 11 while the problems arising from urinary tract disease are considered in Chapter 10. The main source of disorders requiring fluid therapy, however, is gastrointestinal dysfunction and the remainder of this chapter therefore considers the resulting inter-actions between fluid, electrolyte and acid−base disturbances.

Diarrhoea (Figure 2.5)

The faecal losses are sodium and water in varying proportions together with bicarbonate and potassium. Metabolic acidosis is therefore prob-able and may conceal cellular potassium depletion by raising plasma potassium. The loss of sodium and water causes ECF volume contrac-tion and this, in turn, impairs renal function. In mild volume depletion, urinary losses of potassium are accelerated by aldosterone but in severe volume depletion potassium excretion is restricted by inad-equate delivery of sodium to the distal tubule.

Initially, therefore, it is wise to avoid solutions with potassium concentrations above plasma but potassium-free solutions are also inappropriate. During recovery from acidosis, additional potassium may be needed because K^+ can now move from plasma back into cells all the more readily if they have underlying deficits [39]. If the dehydration associated with diarrhoea is severe enough to cause shock, this will intensify the acidosis.

Plasma sodium concentration is essentially subject to three influ-ences which may conflict:

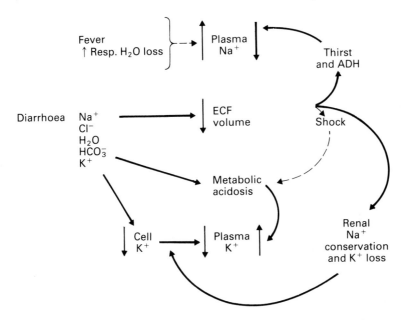

Fig. 2.5 Effects of diarrhoea.

1 The relative loss of sodium and water in faeces.
2 Increased water losses, e.g. due to fever or hyperventilation, especially in warm, dry surroundings.
3 The sustained drive to drinking and renal water retention caused by ECF volume depletion. This causes a strong tendency for plasma Na$^+$ concentration to fall, especially as dietary intake is probably zero, whereas drinking often continues. Correction therefore requires repair of ECF volume, not the provision of hypertonic sodium solutions. Availability of water and encouragement to drink should correct any rises of plasma sodium, provided the animal is not too weak or drinking too painful.

Vomiting and gastric dysfunction (Figure 2.6)

The main loss in vomit is usually hydrochloric acid, i.e. H$^+$ and Cl$^-$, together with water and sodium. There is not a major loss of K$^+$ directly [18], but as ECF volume becomes depleted, the kidney conserves Na$^+$ and urinary potassium losses increase sufficiently to cause K$^+$ depletion [40]. The likely result of vomiting, therefore, is metabolic alkalosis, volume depletion and potassium depletion provided it is

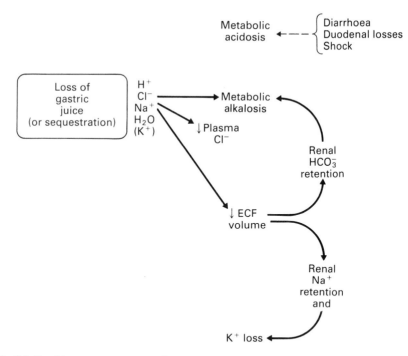

Fig. 2.6 Vomiting or sequestration of gastric juice.

sufficiently sustained or severe. Hypokalaemia is probable as a result of cellular K^+ depletion and alkaline plasma pH (moving K^+ into cells as H^+ exits into plasma) [41]. Abomasal or gastric torsion and dilation can produce similar fluid and electrolyte disturbances by allowing massive accumulation of gastric fluid within the distended viscus [42, 43]; plasma composition suffers even though no external losses occur (see Chapter 9).

Though typical of gastric dysfunction, metabolic alkalosis is not the inevitable outcome. Particularly with torsion and dilatation in dogs, the sequestration of gastric juice within the distended stomach, together with obstruction to venous return and ischaemic damage may be severe enough to cause shock (Chapter 9). There is then a direct conflict between the alkalosis caused by the accumulating fluid and the acidosis caused by shock; the outcome is therefore variable [44, 45]. If vomiting includes substantial quantities of fluid refluxed from the duodenum, typically with heavily bile-stained vomit, there will be loss of alkali as well as acid and again the outcome is variable;

acidosis is possible. Obviously the combination of vomiting with diar-rhoea can readily lead to acidosis rather than alkalosis.

It is clearly possible to make a sound assessment of the probable acid−base disturbance in many cases, based on clinical history, but considerations such as those just discussed suggest that it is usually desirable and sometimes essential to confirm the diagnosis by labora-tory evaluation. The available techniques are outlined in Chapter 5.

References

1 Michell, A.R. (1988) Renal function, renal damage and renal failure. In: *Renal Disease in Dogs and Cats*, 5−29. Michell, A.R. (ed). Blackwell Scientific Publications, Oxford.

2 O'Shaughnessy, W.B. (1831) Letter. *Lancet* **i**, 490.

3 Flear, C.T.G. (1970) Electrolyte and body water changes after trauma. *Journal of Clinical Pathology* (Suppl.) **4**, 16−31.

4 Michell, A.R. (1985) What is shock? *Journal of Small Animal Practice* **26**, 719−38.

5 Michell, A.R. (1988) Diuretics and cardiovascular disease. *Journal of Veterinary Parmacology and Therapeutics* **11**, 246−53.

6 Michell, A.R. (1983) Abnormalities of renal function. In: *Veterinary Nephrology*, 189−210. Hall, L.W. (ed). Heinemann, London.

7 Stanton, R.C., Seifter, J.L. & Brenner, B.M. (1987) Pathogenesis of salt and water retention in congestive heart failure. In: *Body Fluid Homeostasis*, 277−98. Brenner, B.M. & Stein, J.H. (eds). Churchill Livingstone, New York.

8 Epstein, M. (1987) Pathogenesis of sodium retention in liver disease. In: *Body Fluid Homeostasis*, 299−333. Brenner, B.M. & Stein, J.H. (eds). Churchill Livingstone, New York.

9 Carroll, H.J. & Oh, M.S. (1978) Disturbances of body fluid osmolality. *Water, Electrolyte and Acid−Base Metabolism*, 101−43. Lippincott, Philadelphia.

10 Shapiro, J.I. & Anderson, R.J. (1987) Sodium depletion states. In: *Body Fluid Homeostasis*, 245−76. Brenner, B.M. & Stein, J.H. (eds), Churchill Livingstone, New York.

11 Kopple, J.B. & Blumenkrantz, M.J. (1980) Total parenteral nutrition and parenteral fluid therapy. In: *Clinical Disorders of Fluid and Electrolyte Metabolism*, 460−98. Maxwell, M.H. & Kleeman, C.R. (eds). McGraw Hill, New York

12 Michell, A.R. (1979) Biochemistry and behaviour: systemic aspects of neurological disturbance. *Journal of Small Animal Practice* **20**, 645−9.

13 Arieff, A.I. (1988) Central nervous system effects of acute and chronic disturbances of plasma sodium: consequences of rapid v. slow correction. In: *Nephrology*, Vol. 1. 676−87. Davison, A.M. (ed). Bailliere, London.

14 Tyler, R.D., Qualls, C.W., Heald, R.D., Cowell, R.L. & Clinkenbeard, K.D. (1987) Renal function in dogs in with hyponatraemia. *Journal of the American Veterinary Medical Association* **191**, 1095−8.

15 Finberg, L. (1983) Hypernatraemia. In: *Sodium: its Biological Significance*, 266−76. Papper, S. (ed). C.R.C. Press, Florida.

16 Blood, D.C., Radostits, O.M. & Henderson, J.A. (1983) *Veterinary Medicine*, 1116−9. Bailliere Tindall, London.

17 Beck, L.H. (1981) Edema states and the use of diuretics. *Medical Clinics of North America* **65**, 291−302.

18 Lindeman, R.D. & Pederson, J.A. (1983) Hypokalaemia. In: *Potassium: its Biological Significance*, 45−76. Whang, R.H. (ed). C.R.C. Press, Florida.

19 Schaer, M. (1982) Disorders of potassium metabolism. *Veterinary Clinics of North America: Small Animal Practice* **12**, 399−409.

20 Dow, S.W., Le Couteur, R.A., Fettman, M.J. & Spurgeon, T.L. (1987) Potassium depletion in cats: hypokalaemic polymyopathy. *Journal of the American Veterinary Medical Association* **191**, 1563−8.

21 Muylle, E., Nuytten, J., Van den Hende, C., Deprez, P., Vlaminck, K. & Oyaert, W. (1984) Determination of red blood cell potassium content in horses with diarrhoea. *Equine Veterinary Journal* **16**, 450−4.

22 Narins, R.G. (1978) The renal acidoses. In: *Acid−Base and Potassium Homeostasis*, 30−64. Brenner, B.M. & Stein, J.H. (eds). Churchill Livingstone, New York.

23 Carroll, H.J. & Oh, M.S. (1978) *Water, Electrolyte and Acid−Base Metabolism*, 216−305. Lippincott, Philadelphia.

24 Arruda, J.A.L. (1981) Acidosis of renal failure. *Seminars in Nephrology* **1**, 275−80.

25 Michell, A.R. (1970) Protons, pH and survival. *Journal of the American Veterinary Medical Association* **157**, 1540−8.

26 Johnston, D.G. & Alberti, K.G.M. (1983) Acid−base balance in metabolic acidoses. *Clinics in Endocrinology and Metabolism* **12**, 267−85.

27 Sestoft, L. & Bartels, P.D. (1983) Biochemistry and differential diagnosis of metabolic acidoses. *Clinics in Endocrinology and Metabolism* **12**, 287−301.

28 Park, R. & Arieff, A.I. (1983) Lactic acidosis: current concepts. *Clinics in Endocrinology and Metabolism* **12**, 339−58.

29 Cohen, J.J. & Kassirer, J.P. (1982) *Acid−Base*, 385. Little Brown & Co., Boston.

30 Cohen, J.J. & Kassirer, J.P. (1982) *Acid−Base*, 121−226. Little Brown & Co., Boston.

31 Polzin, D.J. & Osborne, C.A. (1986) Anion gap — diagnostic and therapeutic applications. In: *Current Veterinary Therapy* IX, 52−66. Kirk, R.W. (ed). W.B. Saunders, Philadelphia.

32 Groutides, C & Michell, A.R. (1988) A simple, accurate and inexpensive method for assessment of acid−base disturbances in veterinary practice. *Clinical Insight* **3**, 209−10.

33 Rose, B.D. (1977) *Clinical Physiology of Acid−Base and Electrolyte Disorders*, 323−53. McGraw Hill, New York.

34 Hartsfield, S.M., Thurman, J.C. & Benson, G.J. (1981) Sodium bicarbonate and bicarbonate precursors for treatment of metabolic acidosis. *Journal of the American Veterinary Medical Association* **179**, 914−6.

35 Michell, A.R. (1988) Drips, drinks and drenches; what matters in fluid therapy? *Irish Veterinary Journal* **42**, 17−22.

36 Dubose, T.D. (1981) Metabolic alkalosis. *Seminars in Nephrology* **1**, 281−9.

37 Brobst, D. (1986) Pathophysiology of alterations in potassium homeostasis. *Journal of the American Veterinary Medical Association.* **188**, 1019−25.

38 Tannen, R.L. (1987) Effect of potassium on renal acidification and acid−base homeostasis. *Seminars in Nephrology* **7**, 263−73.

39 Oster, J.R. (1981) Metabolic acidosis. *Seminars in Nephrology* **1**, 250−9.

40 Bell, F.W. & Osborne, C.A. (1986) Treatment of hypokalaemia. In: *Current Veterinary Therapy* IX, 101−7. W.B. Saunders, Philadelphia.

41 Sterns, R.H. & Spital, A. (1987) Disorders of internal potassium balance. *Seminars in Nephrology* **7**, 206−22.

42 Gabel, A.A. & Heath, R.B. (1969) Treatment of right-sided torsion of the abomasum in cattle. *Journal of the American Veterinary Medical Association* **155**, 642−4.

43 Winkler, J.K. (1977) Supportive therapy for bovine gastrointestinal stasis and obstruction. *Auburn Veterinarian* (Fall), 7−11.

44 Matthiesen, D.T. (1983) The gastric dilatation-volvulus complex: medical and surgical considerations. *American Animal Hospital Association Journal* **19**, 925−32.

45 Muir, W.M. (1982) Acid−base and electrolyte disturbances in dogs with gastric dilatation-volvulus. *Journal of the American Veterinary Medical Association* **181**, 229−31.

Chapter 3
Composition and choice of fluids

This chapter is concerned with the choice and composition of fluids for oral and parenteral use; the question of oral rehydration is discussed further in Chapter 9.

The intended use of a parenteral fluid can almost invariably be deduced from a comparison of its composition with that of normal plasma (Table 3.1). It is useful to classify the primary purpose of the fluid among the following headings, recognizing that some fluids may fulfil several functions:

1 ECF replacement.
2 Plasma support.
3 ECF alkalinizers.
4 ECF acidifiers.
5 ECF diluent.
6 Maintenance solutions.
7 Nutrient solutions.
8 Concentrated additives.

While a number of specific solutions are referred to, there is no intention to provide a comprehensive list. The central message of this chapter is to encourage confidence in two beliefs; firstly that no formulation need have its function remembered because it is self-evident in the composition. Secondly, that any solution can be modified, if necessary, to improve or change its purpose. The choice of fluids, therefore, is not a mystique, does not require unattainable wisdom nor should it be a ritual — 'we always use x'; literally, for everything.

ECF replacement

Solutions for this purpose must restore ECF volume without distorting ECF composition. Since sodium is the osmotic skeleton of ECF

(Chapter 1) such solutions must, therefore, have a plasma-like concentration of sodium and preferably of chloride and bicarbonate (or its precursors). Volume depletion frequently leads to hyperkalaemia so the K content is preferably not higher than plasma, at least for initial resuscitation but the solution should not be K-free, especially if it yields bicarbonate, because recovery from acidosis may allow development of hypokalaemia (Chapter 2). Calves with diarrhoea are liable to develop hypokalaemia, especially with cessation of oral intake, but dying claves tend to become hyperkalaemic (acidosis, shock, impaired renal function) [1, 2].

The most familiar example of a solution for replacement of ECF volume is Hartmann's lactated Ringer solution. Having a plasma-like concentration of bicarbonate precursor it will improve a mild acidosis, both because it exceeds the bicarbonate content of *acidotic* plasma and, more important, because volume expansion allows improved renal perfusion and thereby restores the ability of the kidney to regulate plasma pH. Thus even 'normal' saline, which is really an ECF acidifier, may improve an acidosis by expanding ECF volume and improving renal (and hepatic) regulation of plasma pH. Normal saline contains somewhat more sodium than plasma, much more chloride and since it is 0.9% (154 mmol/l) it is neither normal physiologically nor chemically.

Darrow's solution, formulated for infant diarrhoea, takes account of the likelihood of potassium depletion and the tendency of children to become hypernatraemic, especially in warm, dry surroundings. In the absence of specific laboratory measurements to justify its use, its lower sodium content and its elevated potassium content are not ideal for the initial treatment of volume depletion. This solution is sometimes described as an 'intracellular rehydrating fluid' [3]. While it is true that the K will mainly reach ICF, this is a misnomer because most of the administered fluid will remain in ECF, held by the Na, which is only a little below plasma concentration. Moreover, even if an animal were to receive 10% of its body weight as Darrow's solution, this would be 3.5 mmol/kg of K compared with an intracellular total of 37 mmol/kg [4], i.e. it could only match a deficit of less than 10% of body K. An animal with a normal plasma pH and a plasma K below 2.3 mmol/l could well have lost over 20% of intracellular K [5]. Thus, while parenteral solutions can be used to defend plasma K, the safest way of providing the large quantities of K needed for intracellular deficits, is orally (Chapter 2).

Table 3.1 Some commercial parenteral solutions (mmol/l)

	Na	K	Cl	Bicarbonate/precursor		Glucose %	Ca^{++}/Mg^{++}
ECF repair							
Ringer acetate	131	5	111	28	Acetate		+/
Hartmann's	131	5	111	28	Lactate		+/
McSherry's	138	12	100	50	Acetate		+/+
Darrow's	121	35	103	53	Lactate		
Normal saline in glucose	154		154	0		5.0	
50% normal saline	77		77	0		2.5	
in glucose	77		77	0		5.0	
Additional alkali							
NaHCO$_3$							
1.4%	167			167			
2.7%	334			334			
4.2%	500			500			
8.4%	1000			1000			
Sodium lactate 1/6 M	167			167	Lactate		
ECF acidifier(see also ECF repair: zero bicarbonate)							
Saline 0.9%	154		154				
Saline 0.9% + KCl	154	27	181				
Ringer's	147	4	156				+/
Additional potassium							
K$_2$HPO$_4$		2000					
KCl		1000–3000					

Colloids					
Haemaccel 3.5%	145	5	150		+/
Dextran 40 or 70 in 0.9% NaCl	150		150		
Dextran 40 or 70 in 5% dextrose				5	
Maintenance					
$\frac{1}{5}$ normal saline (0.18%) in glucose	31		31	4.3	
ECF diluent					
5% glucose				5	
Hypertonic saline e.g. 5% saline	855		855		
Dextrose 5–50%				5–50	
Normal plasma	145	5	100	25	*(for comparison)*

N.B. **1** Minor variants occur even in named solutions.
2 There is a much greater variety of combinations, e.g. of KCl–glucose or KCl–saline, or glucose–saline.

Plasma support

Just as albumin allows plasma to maintain its volume despite the hydrostatic pressure tending to drive water out of the capillaries (Chapter 1) solutions with molecules large enough to be retained within capillaries specifically boost plasma volume, rather than interstitial volume. Such solutions, 'colloids', will be retained in plasma and if they are hypertonic, they will draw in additional fluid from the interstitial compartment. The colloid thus allows the associated electrolyte solution to be retained in circulation. Obviously a pure electrolyte solution (crystalloid) can boost plasma volume just as effectively as a colloid but much more is needed because the majority distributes into interstitial fluid — this tends to offset the fact that crystalloids are less expensive. On the other hand the traditional idea that colloids are less likely to cause pulmonary oedema now seems dubious (Chapter 4) because elevation of venous pressure, rather than dilution of plasma proteins, appears to be the critical factor. Thus over-rapid administration of colloids, since they remain intravascular, will cause pulmonary oedema. Equally, over-treatment with crystalloids will cause oedema by lowering the plasma protein concentration [6, 7]. The crystalloid versus colloid debate cannot yet be resolved even in human medicine because 'a lot of frequently cited work do not rest on very firm ground — rather like the debate about corticosteroids in shock' [8]. The nature of the debate should be emphasized; however, there is no doubt that, volume for volume, colloids give more effective repair of *plasma* volume. The controversy surrounds the traditional idea that they are less likely to cause pulmonary oedema if used in excess.

Blood and its derivatives (e.g. plasma) are colloids but they are considered in Chapter 8. Here we are concerned with artificial colloids notably dextrans, gelatin and hydroxyethyl starch. Although these can substitute for the effect of albumin in preserving blood volume, the effect is temporary and they do not substitute for the transport functions of albumin; moreover they may depress its synthesis [7].

Dextrans are artificial carbohydrates similar to 'sephadex' (used as a biochemical separating medium). They come in a variety of molecular weights, the two remaining in common use being 70 and 40, with predominant molecular weights of 70 000 and 40 000 respectively (each contains a range of molecular weights). With a molecular weight close to albumin, dextran 70 is retained well in circulation whereas dextran 40 only survives about a quarter as long and may cause osmotic diuresis [9]. Dextran 40, however, with its smaller molecular weight, is more osmotically active and is usually provided in a hypertonic preparation. This draws fluid into capillaries from interstitial fluid, coats red cells and endothelium and thus improves capillary flow, breaking up microaggregates, and helping to counter the problems of capillary perfusion associated with shock (Chapter 3).

Dextrans have some problems [10, 11]. Firstly, they can be antigenic, especially those with larger molecular weights (notably those above 100000 which are almost extinct). By coating red cells, they interfere with cross matching of blood (but this is seldom done in veterinary practice and a sample can be taken before administration). They also interfere with haemostasis but this risk exists with any artificial colloid used in excess and the volume used should not exceed 20% of estimated normal blood volume [11]. More recent evidence suggests that interference with blood typing only occurs at higher concentrations [12]. Dextran 40, in particular, can precipitate acute renal failure but, like hypersensitivity, this problem is only likely to occur in a very small proportion of individuals. Horses may be more prone to hypersensitivity especially with repeated use but this seems to be a clinical impression rather than an accurately documented statistic [13]. It is possible to do an intradermal test for hypersensitivity and it is also possible to protect against it by prior injection of a much lower molecular weight dextran (1000) [14].

Gelatin of bovine origin, suitably treated to eliminate its antigenicity, 'Haemaccel', is probably the most popular colloid in veterinary use in the UK. It is claimed to have less side effects than dextran, notably hypersensitivity and anticoagulation, but having half the average molecular weight, it does not persist as effectively as Dextran 70 (around 3 hours, as opposed to 8–10 hours) nor does it have the particular virtues of Dextran 40 [12, 15–17]. There have not been clinical trials which would really permit a comparison of the effectiveness and untoward effects of these colloids in veterinary practice; moreover their persistence in circulation varies with the hydration of the animal, so that comparisons require caution. Generally, artificial colloids are less effective than albumin, because being uncharged, they exert less osmotic effect [18]. The choice remains a matter of personal judgement and experience. Dextran has the reputation with some veterinarians of giving a more slippery texture to blood and therefore making surgical manipulation more difficult. The problem of side effects should not be exaggerated; the risk with dextran in humans is about 1 in 3000 and is slightly greater with gelatin preparations [12]. 'Gelafusin' is another gelatin-based colloid.

Hydroxyethyl starch (HES) [19, 19a], 'Volex' has been hovering in the human literature for many years but despite certain advantages, e.g. fewer side effects, it has failed to displace existing materials. Although its molecular weight is much higher than Dextran 70, it is a much more compact molecule and has a similar osmotic effect. It persists slightly longer and produces less hypersensitivity reaction. Its veterinary impact has been almost zero. Nevertheless, it is worth mentioning because current research with artificial bloods utilizes fluorocarbons as oxygen carriers and HES as the colloid [20]. While existing products are unsatisfactory in that they only work in an enriched oxygen atmosphere, further development may considerably influence veterinary medicine and reduce the problems of blood banking (Chapter 8). There is a strong drive to develop artificial blood for human use because blood itself is not only scarce but, as a result of hepatitis and AIDS, it has become a hazardous material.

ECF alkalinizers

These contain bicarbonate, or a precursor such as lactate or acetate (Chapter 2). Hartmann's (lactated Ringer) solution is relatively safe in that it yields more bicarbonate than the concentration in acidotic plasma but no more than normal plasma. Acetated Ringer solution is less dependent on liver for its utilization [21] and would certainly be preferable in an acidotic animal known to have liver disease. A number of solutions contain the additional amount of bicarbonate (or precursor) required to correct a severe acidosis, e.g. McSherry's or Rose's solution (Table 3.1), and they frequently have more K since the improvement of an acidosis usually (but not invariably) lowers plasma K (Chapter 2). Manufacturers tend to favour precursors rather than bicarbonate because they are easier to sterilize and have fewer drug incompatibilities [22]. In addition, the gradual yield gives a greater margin of safety. The adverse effects of excess bicarbonate will be initially to cause persistent hyperventilation in animals recovering from metabolic acidosis (Chapter 2), to reduce liberation of oxygen from haemoglobin, to depress plasma potassium and free-calcium and ultimately to depress respiration [23, 24]. *Some* commercial Hartmann's solutions contain phenolic preservatives such as methylparaben which make them dangerous for cats [25].

ECF acidifiers

It is possible to acidify ECF and thus treat metabolic alkalosis with HCl or more usually with NH_4Cl which yields HCl once it is metabolized. Much more simply, however, 'normal' saline provides a bicarbonate-free expansion of ECF, rich in chloride and is therefore an excellent treatment for metabolic alkalosis. Ringer's solution acts similarly but contains some additional ions, notably K (Table 3.1). The important point, frequently forgotten, is that it is not the same as Hartmann's solution, its lactated derivative.

ECF diluent

It is convenient to have a means of supplying water intravenously, if necessary, without causing osmotic shock to red cells. This is achieved by giving it in a temporarily isotonic form, namely 5% glucose. The glucose is metabolized and the net result is provision of water. The calorie yield of 5% glucose is pitiful but it can provide a transient defence against hypoglycaemia. In solution, 1 g of glucose yields 3.4 kcal [9] and since the maintenance requirement exceeds 50 kcal (210 kJ)/kg/day, it would take over 5 l/day to supply a 20 kg dog. Hence nutritional support requires more concentrated solutions (see Chapter 12).

Maintenance solutions

These are intended to substitute for normal drinking and for the major electrolytes contained in food, i.e. they are used to offset the effects of anorexia persisting beyond a day or two, and of inadequate fluid intake. The ratio of sodium to water requirement results in a solution with about 20% of the sodium content of plasma (N/5) and maintenance solutions generally contain similar concentrations of other electrolytes (i.e. below 30 mmol/l), notably potassium. Although they are frequently given subcutaneously they are meant exclusively for intravenous use [26, 27] and should certainly not be used subcutaneously in a clearly dehydrated animal. The reason is that the subcutaneous pool of dilute saline will initially attract sodium out of circulation and thus diminish plasma volume before it is eventually absorbed. These solutions typically have sufficient glucose to make them isotonic, i.e. since they already contain electrolytes the glucose content is even less than 5%. In no sense, therefore, do they provide nutritional maintenance, i.e. adequate supplies of calories (or nitrogen).

Nutrient solutions

Since the late 1940s techniques have been available to allow the total intravenous nutritional maintenance of dogs and subsequently humans [28, 29]. Thus gut can be 'rested' when appropriate or its function can be substituted until it recovers, even over many weeks or months. Bypass of the gut, in favour of intravenous nutrition, however, is not without adverse effect on the intestine itself since it has a rapid turnover of cells and rapidly readjusts its form to its function [30]. Moreover, since these solutions are both concentrated and highly nutritive they combine the tendency to irritate veins with the ability to foster bacterial proliferation [31]. The major problem (and expense) therefore, is the supervision of the i.v. access itself. Unfortunately, infusions need to be given over an extended period since if glucose is supplied too fast (over 0.5 g/kg/hour) [32] it merely spills into urine by exceeding the maximum rate of renal reabsorption. A variety of solutions exist, based on concentrated glucose, alcohol or lipid emulsion for calories and protein hydrolysates or synthetic amino acid mixtures (very expensive) for nitrogen [33]. With more extended dependence on total parenteral nutrition, attention to trace elements and vitamins as well as major electrolytes becomes important [34]. The subject of total parenteral nutrition (TPN) is considered in more detail in Chapter 12. Despite its canine origin it has, so far, had little veterinary impact.

Concentrated additives

These are usually solutions of single salts, e.g. sodium bicarbonate or potassium chloride, which are intended to boost the content of another solution and are therefore extremely concentrated (e.g. 1 mmol/ml). Thus, addition of 25 ml of 8.4% bicarbonate (1 mmol/ml) to a litre of Hartmann's solution would virtually double its eventual bicarbonate yield (and also raise its sodium, like that of 'normal saline' somewhat above plasma). The error in ignoring the additional volume is negligible (less than 1 mmol/l in this example). Such concentrated solutions should never be administered directly to an animal. This can happen unintentionally, however, for example if KCl is added to a plastic drip pack and no effort is made to mix it. The added potassium may form a layer beneath the rest of the solution and enter the animal at virtually 1 mmol/ml, with euthanasia the likely result!

Sodium bicarbonate is also available as 4.2% and as 1/6 M (1.4%) which though approximately isotonic (slightly hypertonic) is far above plasma bicarbonate concentration. Sodium lactate is also available as a 1/6 M solution. Both contain 167 mmol/l of bicarbonate (or precursor) and sodium and if used 1:3 with Hartmann's solution the result is a mixture with a sodium concentration closer to plasma (140 mmol/l) and 2.25 times the bicarbonate yield of Hartmann's itself. Rose [35] has suggested that the addition of 60 mmol of sodium bicarbonate and 20 mmol of KCl to each litre of N/2 saline provides an excellent repair solution for acidosis having Na 137, K 20, Cl 97 and bicarbonate 60; the additional K is to take account of cell uptake during recovery.

Treatment of hyperkalaemia

Once plasma potassium concentration exceeds 7 mmol/l it becomes a matter of some urgency to reduce it before cardiac function is impaired [36]. There are essentially three approaches. [37, 38]:

1 To drive potassium into cells by treating any acidosis and by using a combination of glucose and insulin to promote active uptake.

2 To oppose the adverse effects of K, by injecting calcium borogluconate.

3 To promote potassium excretion using oral ion exchange resins or, in an extreme emergency, peritoneal dialysis.

Recently, the first of these approaches has been extended by experimental use of β_2 agonists (e.g. salbutamol) to drive K^+ into cells [39].

Hypertonic saline

It is possible to obtain hypertonic saline solutions (e.g. 3%, 5%; 513, 855 mmol/l) but since hyponatraemia is usually corrected by restoration of ECF volume (Chapter 2), and sometimes by water restriction, there are very few indications for such solutions. Moreover, since plasma sodium concentration is not readily monitored in most practice laboratories, their use is potentially hazardous. A quite separate use for small volumes of hypertonic saline, for effects other than those on plasma Na or ECF volume, has emerged in the treatment of shock and is discussed in Chapter 4.

Components of therapy

The main concern in fluid therapy is the correction of existing deficits, 'deficit therapy'. In addition, during periods of reduced food and fluid intake the use of maintenance solutions may become necessary (see above), tapering off as normal intake is resumed, 'maintenance therapy'. Finally, since abnormal losses may continue during treatment, consideration has to be given to their replacement, 'contemporary loss therapy'. Ideally, this takes account of the composition of the losses but more often it has to take the form of an additional allowance in the deficit therapy (Chapter 6). Thus, any regimen for fluid therapy should consider the demands of deficit, contemporary loss or maintenance therapy [40, 41] even if all three do not require provision in every case, or if contemporary loss and deficit therapy are merged in a single infusion. The aim of deficit therapy is not the immediate correction of the entire calculated deficit. Rather, the objective is ideally to replace half the deficit in the first 6 hours, three-quarters during the first 24 hours and to complete deficit therapy in the first 48 hours. This allows ample opportunity to monitor the response to therapy both clinically and with whatever serial laboratory estimations are available (Chapter 5). It is thus possible to revise the initial assessment in the light of progress and, in particular, to avoid the adverse effects of over-treatment if the initial estimates of deficit turn out to be high.

The application of these principles to the design of therapy for specific clinical conditions and the combined disturbances which they present is illustrated in subsequent chapters.

Oral rehydration

Oral rehydration (Table 3.2) is discussed in greater detail in the context of gastrointestinal disturbances (Chapter 9). It is an excellent method of rehydration provided the fluid does not cause vomiting,

Table 3.2 Some oral rehydration solutions

	Na	K	Cl	Bicarbonate/ precursor		Glucose %	Ca+Mg	Other
Ionalyte	155	12	106	61	Acetate	0	+	
IRT	140	10	103	74	Acetate	0	+	
Electrosol	138	8	83	68	Acetate	2.5	+	
Zawbolyte	192	13	71	32	Acetate	0	+	Attapulgite
Volac anti-scour	27	5	21	11		0.75	Mg	Organic pulp
Enterolyte	1472	90	883	734	Acetate	0	+	Antibiotics, etc.
Daltons*	42	26	39	21		5.0		PO_4
WHO-type formulations								
Beecham scour	73	16	73	2	Citrate	2.2		Glycine, PO_4
Lectade	73	16	73	2	Citrate	2.2		Glycine, PO_4
Lectade plus	50	20	39	29†	Citrate	3.1		Glycine, PO_4
Life aid	76	15	74	2	Propionate	2		Glycine, PO_4
Ion aid	75	26	75	0		2.1	+	Glycine
Electydral	80	25	54	50	Acetate + Propionate	1.5	Mg	

The composition shown is the approximate concentration (mmol/l) received by the animal if the solution is made up as directed (modified from [27]).

* Non-commercial.

† 1 mmol of citrate = 3 mmol bicarbonate.

the animal is not collapsed or shocked, and oral fluids are not contraindicated. It is a particularly safe route for the repair of potassium deficits.

In assessing the probable usefulness of an oral rehydration solution (ORS) the issue is *not* to compare with plasma but with the concentration and formulation most likely to promote intestinal uptake of salt and water. Based on the original research underlying the World Health Organization (WHO) solution for the treatment of cholera (and subsequently many other forms of diarrhoea), something of the order of an equimolar sodium and glucose solution which was also isotonic seemed ideal, i.e.

2% glucose (100 mmol/l)

Na^+ (100 mmol/l)

Cl^- and other anions (100 mmol/l).

Subsequently the main areas of discussion have been [42]:

1 Whether sodium should be reduced for fear of hypernatraemia. This fear seems misplaced, and the less sodium absorbed, the less ECF volume can be replaced.

2 Whether the anions should include a source of bicarbonate. If the condition causes metabolic acidosis, as is often the case, this is desirable since the solution will provide a more effective repair. Otherwise repair of the acidosis depends solely on improved renal function associated with restoration of circulating volume. Precursors (e.g. citrate, acetate) also help sodium uptake and, unlike bicarbonate, do not undermine gastric acidity, thereby increasing susceptibility to enteric pathogens.

3 Whether the calorie content can be higher, i.e. the glucose concentration increased. The benefit is to avoid hypoglycaemia, especially in young animals, since the optimal ORS formulation for absorption is inescapably inadequate as a sole source of calories. The risk is of causing hypernatraemia (by making the solution hypertonic and drawing water into the gut) or of causing further diarrhoea through malabsorption and fermentation of the additional sugar. There are, as yet, few definitive answers, i.e. based on clinical trials in specified conditions and in species of primary veterinary concern. In calves with diarrhoea, however, there is evidence to suggest that a greater glucose concentration is beneficial [42].

References

1 Groutides, C.P. (1988) Studies of fluid, electrolyte and acid−base balance in diarrhoeic calves with special reference to fluid therapy. PhD Thesis, University of London.

2 Phillips, R.W. & Lewis, L.D. (1980) Intravenous high potassium therapy for diarrhoeic calves. *Proceedings of the XIth International Congress on Diseases of Cattle, Tel Aviv*, Vol. II, 1529−35.

3 Clark, C.H. (1981) Fluid therapy. In: *Veterinary Critical Care*, 415−34. Sattler, F.D., Knowles, R.P. & Whittick, W.G. (eds). Lea & Febiger, Philadelphia.

4 Carroll, H.J. & Oh, M.S. (1978) *Water, Electrolyte and Acid−Base Metabolism*, 9. J.B. Lippincott, Philadelphia.

5 Haskins, S. (1984) Fluid and electrolyte therapy. *Compendium of Continuing Education for the Practising Veterinarian* **6**, 244−54.

6 Moss, G.S., Lowe, R.J., Jilek, J. & Levine, H.D. (1982) Fluid therapy in shock. In: *Massive Transfusion in Surgery and Trauma*, 51−63. Collins, J.A., Murawski, K. & Shafer, A.W. (eds). Alan Liss, New York.

7 Blauhut, B.B. & Lundsgaard-Hansen, P. (1986) *Albumin and the Systemic Circulation*, 18−36, 86−100, 155−76, 186−98. Karger, Basel.

8 Suter, P.M. (1986) In: *Albumin and the Systemic Circulation*, 199−202. Karger, Basel.

9 Kopple, J.D. & Blumenkrantz, M.J. (1980) In: *Clinical Disorders of Fluid and Electrolyte Metabolism*, 482−6. Maxwell, M.H. & Kleeman, C.R. (eds). McGraw Hill, New York.

10 Willatts, S. M. (1987) *Lecture Notes on Fluid and Electrolyte Balance*, 240−1. Blackwell Scientific Publications, Oxford.

11 Michell, A.R. (1979) Fluid therapy: some specific applications to medical conditions in small animals. *Veterinary Record* **104**, 572−5.

12 Lutz, H. & Georgieff, M. (1986) In: *Albumin and the Systemic Circulation*, 145−54. Blauhut, B.B. & Lundsgaard-Hansen, P. (eds). Karger, Basel.

13 Carlson, G.P. (1979) Fluid therapy in horses with acute diarrhoea. *Veterinary Clinics of North America: Large Animal Practice* **1**, 313−29.

14 Demling, R.H. (1986) In: *Albumin and the Systemic Circulation*, 36−52. Blauhut, B.B. & Lundsgaard-Hansen, P (eds). Karger, Basel.

15 Isbister, J.P. & Fisher, M.M. (1980) Adverse effects of plasma volume expanders. *Anaesthesia and Intensive Care* **8**, 145−51.

16 Chien, S., Dormandy, J., Ernst, E. & Matrai, A. (1987) In: *Clinical Hemorheology*, 311−38. Chien, S. Dormandy, J. Ernst, E. & Matsai, A (eds). Martinus Nijhoff, Amsterdam.

17 Yoxall, A.T. (1980) Acute circulatory failure — shock. In: *Physiological Basis of Small Animal Medicine*, 201−3. Yoxall, A.T. & Hird, J.F.R. (eds). Blackwell Scientific Publications, Oxford.

18 Veech, R.L. (1986) The toxic impact of parenteral solutions on the metabolism of cells. *American Journal of Clinical Nutrition* **44**, 519−51.

19 Messmer, K. (1984) Blood substitutes in shock therapy. In: *Shock and Related Problems*, 192−205. Shires, G.T. (ed). Churchill Livingstone, New York.

19a Michell, A.R. (1989) Shock in companion animals. In: *Veterinary Annual 29*, Grunsell, C.S.G. & Hill, F.W.G. (eds).

20 Canizaro, P.C. (1984) Oxygen transport. In: *Shock and Related Problems*, 95−110. Shires, G.T. (ed). Churchill Livingstone, New York.

21 Hartsfield, S.M., Thurmon, J.C. & Benson, G.J. (1981) Sodium bicarbonate and bicarbonate precursors for treatment of metabolic acidosis. *Journal of the American Veterinary Medical Association* **179**, 914−16.

22 Michell, A.R. (1983) Fluid therapy for alimentary disease: origins and objectives. *Annales de Recherches Veterinaires* **14**, 527−32.

23 Oster, J.R. (1981) Metabolic acidosis. *Seminars in Nephrology* **1**, 250−9.

24 Park, R. & Arieff, A.I. (1983) Lactic acidosis: current concepts. In: *Metabolic Acidosis*, 339−58. Schade, D.S. (ed). W.B. Saunders, Philadelphia.

25 Keen, P. & Livingston, A. (1983) Adverse reactions to drugs. *In Practice* **5**, 174−80.

26 Gross, D.R. (1985) General concepts of fluid therapy. In: *Veterinary Pharmacology and Therapeutics*, 480−91. Booth, N.H. & McDonald, L.E. (eds). Iowa State University Press, Ames.

27 Michell, A.R. (1983) Understanding fluid therapy. *Irish Veterinary Journal* **37**, 94−103.

28 Michell, A.R. (1979) The pathophysiological basis of fluid therapy in small animals. *Veterinary Record* **104**, 542−8.

29 Li, A.K.C., Wills, M.R. & Hanson, G.R. (1980) *Fluid, Electrolytes, Acid−Base and Nutrition*. Academic Press, London.

30 Levin, R.J. (1984) Intestinal adaptation to dietary change as exemplified by dietary restriction studies. In: *Function and Dysfunction of the Small Intestine*, 77−93. Batt, R. & Lawrence, T. (eds). Liverpool University Press, Liverpool.

31 Lewis, L.D. Morris, M.L. & Hand, M.S. (1987) *Small Animal Clinical Nutrition III*, 5:35−43. Mark Morris Associates, Topeka.

32 Finco, D.R. (1972) General guidelines for fluid therapy. *Journal of the American Animal Hospital Association* **8**, 166−77.

33 Lee, H.A. (1974) Intravenous nutrition. *British Journal of Hospital Medicine* **11**, 719−24.

34 Heatley, R.V. & Tredree, R. (1986) Intravenous feeding. In: *Clinical Nutrition in Gastroenterology*, 117—29. Heatley, R.V., Losowsky, M.S. & Kelleher, J. (eds). Churchill Livingstone, Edinburgh.

35 Rose, R.J. (1981) A physiological approach to fluid and electrolyte therapy in the horse. *Equine Veterinary Journal* **13**, 7—14.

36 Schaer, M. (1982) Disorders of potassium metabolism. *Veterinary Clinics of North America: Small Animal Practice* **12**, 399—409.

37 Kaufman, C.E. & Papper, S. (1983) Hyperkalaemia. In: *Potassium: Its Biologic Significance*, 77—95. Whang, R.D. (ed). C.R.C. Press, Boca Raton, Florida.

38 Silver, M.R. (1985) Disorders of potassium balance. In: *Disorders of Fluid and Electrolyte Balance*, 39—51. Puschett, J.B. & Greenberg, A.G. (eds). Churchill Livingstone, New York.

39 Montoliu, J., Lens, X.M. & Revert, L. (1987) Potassium-lowering effect of albuterol for hyperkalaemia in renal failure. *Archives of Internal Medicine* **147**, 713—7.

40 Cornelius, L.M. (1980) Fluid therapy in small animal practice. *Journal of the American Veterinary Medical Association* **176**, 109—14.

41 Schall, W.D. (1982) General principles of fluid therapy. *Veterinary Clinics of North America: Small Animal Practice* **12**, 453—65.

42 Michell, A.R. (1988) Drips, drinks and drenches: what matters in fluid therapy? *Irish Veterinary Journal* **42**, 17—22.

Chapter 4 _____
Volume depletion and shock

Introduction

The renal defence against volume depletion eventually undermines the regulation of plasma composition, as already described. The circulatory response to volume depletion is also primarily defensive but is similarly achieved only at a cost. These costs become severe as they mount up in the self-reinforcing interactions which lead to circulatory shock. The consequences are widespread and potentially lethal and will ultimately defy correction by replacement of circulating volume alone. Nevertheless, timely volume replacement and an understanding of the underlying pathophysiology remain the principal prerequisites for the successful prevention or treatment of shock. What follows is a summary of the main problems and their origins; for additional references the reader should consult more detailed accounts [1–3].

Vascular effects

Shock is a caricature of the physiological response to haemorrhage; the outline of the defensive features remains recognizable but it is exaggerated and distorted to a degree which becomes both absurd and damaging.

Benefits (Figure 4.1)

The crucial component of the response is vasoconstriction, especially of arterioles. This helps to maintain arterial pressure (upstream) but drops capillary pressure (downstream). As a result it is easier for interstitial fluid to re-enter capillaries, attracted by the osmotic pull of plasma proteins. The smaller component of ECF (plasma) thus receives an internal transfusion from the larger volume in the tissue spaces. This explains the fall in PCV which follows haemorrhage but the

55

(a)

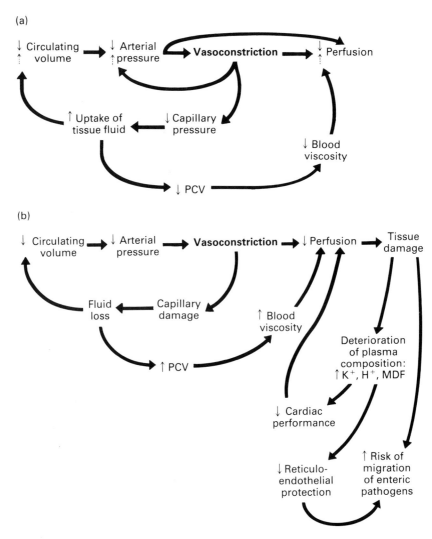

(b)

Fig. 4.1 Vasoconstriction: adverse and beneficial effects; (a) defence against loss of circulating volume; (b) some of the vicious cycles of shock.

effect on tissue oxygenation is unexpected. It requires considerable work to move red cells through capillaries so the more there are, the greater the viscosity of blood, especially if the RBC lose their elasticity and adhere to one another or to capillary walls. By reducing viscosity, haemodilution improves oxygen delivery (Fig. 4.2) which is probably optimal in dogs at a PCV around 30 and little worse at 20 than in

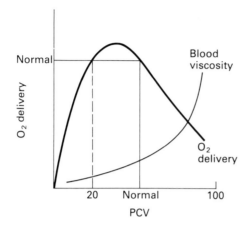

Fig. 4.2 Haematocrit, oxygen delivery and blood viscosity.

normality [4, 5]. In many species including dogs, sheep, humans and horses, splenic contraction can provide an additional boost to the RBC count and limit the fall in PCV. As Wooldridge (1891) perceived, the key to perfusion is not the presence of blood in capillaries but its efficient movement through them; after a haemorrhage there is usually still enough haemoglobin to sustain life 'if only enough fluid could be added to keep it in circulation' [6]. Figure 4.2 illustrates this principle, not specific data, which, in any case, would vary with species. Nevertheless, the principle is an important one: a *high* viscosity gives good oxygen carrying *capacity* but poor *delivery* because the blood is too viscous to flow freely through capillaries. The initial effect of mild haemodilution is to *improve* delivery — which probably only becomes subnormal at a PVC below 20. Perfusion is not about presence (of blood or haemoglobin) but *flow*.

There is also constriction of veins which not only provides a transient boost to venous return (and so to cardiac output) but also transfers a greater proportion of the remaining blood volume from the low pressure storage (venous) side of the system to the high pressure delivery (arterial) side. Above all, it reduces the volume of the system to be filled from a diminished volume of blood. This is reinforced by the combined effects of arteriolar and precapillary sphincter constriction, so reducing the perfusion of an increasingly wide range of 'less essential' capillary beds. Even in normality, the key role of the autonomic nervous system in coordinating circulatory function is to apportion the distribution of a limited supply of blood to a potentially enormous volume of vessels, according to current tissue requirements. A total failure could theoretically allow the entire supply to disappear into the capillaries of the liver alone. In shock the problems are intensified by the diminished volume of blood, the need to encroach on the essential perfusion requirements of important tissues and (in endotoxin shock) the exaggerated perfusion of some capillary beds.

These problems are not soluble without volume replacement and if it is delayed other problems ensue until replacement even with volumes of fluid greatly exceeding the losses will still not restore normality. Moreover, blood may no longer be the ideal replacement fluid, granted the abnormal circulatory system to which it is administered [7]. In fact, particularly if it is badly stored, it can be lethal and prone to coagulation.

Adverse consequences (Figure 4.1)

The acute response to haemorrhage activates a negative feedback system protecting both arterial pressure and circulating volume. The stimulus is a fall in volume and pressure; vasoconstriction corrects both, the latter almost instantaneously. As shock becomes established, the stability of negative feedback is replaced by positive feedback or vicious cycles; the responses amplify the disturbances instead of correcting them.

Eventually vasoconstriction will cause damage not only to under-perfused tissues but to the capillaries themselves. The result is a further fall in circulating volume; positive feedback. It is reinforced by a rise in capillary pressure resulting from venous constriction; this augments the fluid loss and is thus a further vicious cycle. Moreover, the remaining blood in leaky capillaries will have an enhanced PCV and, therefore, a greater viscosity. These problems are compounded by the effects of hypoxia and accumulating metabolites, which increase red cell rigidity and reduce the natural charge repulsion between adjacent red cells and also the surrounding capillary endothelium. Engorgement of capillaries with stagnant RBC becomes a major problem in established shock. In fact, the various adverse changes in capillary perfusion are the most consistent feature of circulatory shock; it is, above all, a failure of the microcirculation.

As shock progresses, the trend towards fluid loss from capillaries (rather than the earlier beneficial uptake) is reinforced by the relaxation of precapillary sphincters under the influence of accumulating metabolites. The venous side is more resistant, thus capillary pressure is raised and promotes further fluid loss. In the advanced stages, there is relaxation of venous outflow but the result is to restore access to a much larger volume of vessels without sufficient blood to maintain an adequate arterial pressure. This becomes an important factor in the terminal stages of shock.

Increased viscosity is not the only feature of blood which deteriorates during shock and so contributes to the problems. Underperfusion of tissues leads to accumulation of metabolites, including H^+ and K^+ and generation of toxic mediators including, probably, kinins, certain prostaglandins, histamine, etc. Even well perfused tissues such as the heart, therefore, suffer from the abnormal composition of the plasma which they receive.

It is familiar and logical that the products of damage to tissues, capillaries or RBC promote clotting and are thus likely to accelerate local haemostasis. Such a response is less logical when excessive vasoconstriction, rather than local trauma, is the cause of the tissue damage and when dehydration, rather than haemorrhage, is the cause of volume depletion. The result can reach two extremes. The first is dissemination of small clots to hitherto unimpeded capillary beds. Eventually, consumption of the precursors for clotting becomes excessive and at the other extreme it prevents adequate coagulation in response to clot displacement and further haemorrhage. Disseminated intravascular coagulation (DIC) thus leads to 'consumptive coagulopathy' [8].

Almost all the problems described so far are direct or indirect results of excessive vasoconstriction and thus of α-adrenergic activity whether associated with sympathetic nerves or circulating adrenaline. Since this is a defensive response made damaging by its intensity, any attempt to remedy it will have potentially harmful, as well as beneficial effects. This is a recurrent theme in the treatment of shock. By relieving vasoconstriction, α-blockers can certainly improve perfusion but they can also be lethal if the underlying stimulus for vasoconstriction, namely volume depletion, is not corrected first. Similarly, the hypotension which may become serious in advanced shock, requires treatment by replacement of circulating volume or improvement of cardiac output.

Cardiac effects

Although the main circulatory problems of shock involve the vessels and the blood (peripheral circulatory failure), the heart also becomes involved, both in the causes and the effects. Cardiac output is usually (but not invariably) depressed in shock, partly because of reduced venous return (peripheral pooling of blood) but also because of impaired performance. The sympatho-adrenal responses accelerate heart rate. Excessive tachycardia, by encroaching on diastole, restricts the time available both for ventricular filling and also for effective myocardial perfusion. There is thus a risk of myocardial hypoxia and this, combined with acidosis, can lead to cardiac damage [1]. Anaesthesia provides additional factors depressing cardiac function and these are reinforced by volume depletion [1, 9].

Recently, much interest has centred on a more specific cause of impaired cardiac performance in shock. Splanchnic vasoconstriction, particularly through its damaging effects on the pancreas, liberates a number of toxic substances into the circulation; one of these potently and specifically depresses cardiac function (myocardial depressant factor, MDF) [2]. Thus, pancreatic damage is both a result and a cause of shock and the presence of MDF not only reduces cardiac output but leads to further compensatory vasoconstriction, perpetuating the vicious cycle (Fig. 4.3).

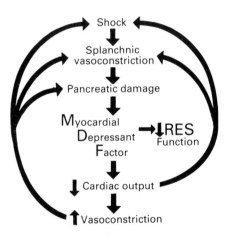

Fig. 4.3 Splanchnic constriction, pancreatic damage and cardiac output.

Splanchnic effects

Apart from causing pancreatic damage, splanchnic vasoconstriction can cause capillary damage in the intestine [10, 11] and thus allow leakage from an enormous surface area. The damage can be sufficiently severe for shock to cause further loss of whole blood within the gut. Secretion of protective mucus is reduced by ischaemia and this, combined with gut stasis, may allow proliferation and invasion by pathogens. The risk of bacterial infection after trauma, therefore, does not simply depend on obvious contamination of wounds. Moreover, reticuloendothelial function is depressed by MDF or a very similar substance [10, 12] and this combines with the effects of reduced hepatic blood flow to increase the animal's vulnerability to bacteria or toxins originating from the gut.

Acidosis

Impairment of hepatic function has an additional important effect; it intensifies the metabolic acidosis caused by shock. Tissue hypoxia not only generates additional H^+, it particularly causes accumulation of lactic acid [13]. Normally, the liver has an ample capacity to metabolize lactate and regenerate bicarbonate [14] but only if it is sufficiently perfused (Chapter 1). The use of lactate as a convenient pharmaceutical precursor [15] for bicarbonate thus rests on adequate hepatic function and the restoration of adequate perfusion by the solution in which it is included. Other precursors such as acetate may well find favour since they do not accumulate in plasma during shock and are more widely utilized outside the liver [16]. Since acetate, for example, is mainly metabolized by muscle [17], which is also subject to vasoconstriction, these anions should perhaps be regarded as additional, rather than alternative precursors. Moreover, they should be used with caution since there is less experience of their effects and, in humans, concern about toxicity, though mainly at high concentration [18].

Pulmonary aspects: shock lung

The most serious adverse effect of excessive (i.e. over-rapid) fluid therapy is pulmonary oedema but shock, or its causes, can also increase pulmonary fluid accumulation. There is thus considerable confusion over the factors contributing to pulmonary oedema after trauma and, in particular, the relative merits of pure electrolyte solutions (crystalloids) compared with colloids [1, 2].

Post-traumatic pulmonary insufficiency was first recognized over 30 years ago, but has become more commonly recognized only relatively recently as resuscitation therapy has improved initial survival rates. Respiratory failure is often the ultimate cause of death in animals which survive the original insult or trauma. The syndrome frequently develops several days after the original trauma. There are numerous theories as to its cause but in truth, several factors are probably involved. Sepsis, fluid overload, DIC, fat emboli, microaggregates and neurogenic factors have all been implicated. The result is a progressive syndrome of dyspnoea, hypoxia and eventually pulmonary oedema. Once established, the syndrome is rapidly progressive and often fatal unless aggressive treatment is instituted.

Colloids are preferable at least for part of the volume replacement in shock (up to 20% of blood volume [4, 19]) because they are retained in plasma and hold accompanying fluids in circulation. Crystalloids equilibrate throughout the ECF and therefore mostly boost interstitial volume rather than plasma. It therefore takes a greater volume to repair the plasma deficit. Initially this does no harm because the interstitial compartment has usually been depleted, partly by capillary uptake in defence of plasma volume. Large volumes of crystalloid, however, can sufficiently dilute plasma proteins to reverse this flow and cause expansion of interstitial fluid, i.e. oedema. Most oedema is merely inconvenient but pulmonary oedema is potentially lethal. The importance of some degree of myocardial oedema in shock [20] may underlie some of the beneficial effects of hyperosmotic solutions in the treatment of shock [1].

Until recently it was thought that excess crystalloid clearly carried a greater risk of causing pulmonary oedema. The forces governing capillary exchange in the lungs, however, are different from those in other tissues (see Fig. 1.3), mainly because the pulmonary arterial pressure is lower. In particular, pulmonary interstitial fluid is relatively rich in protein and this provides an automatic protection against oedema. Accumulation of additional fluid dilutes the interstitial protein and so improves the osmotic gradient for return of fluid to plasma. Apart from capillary damage, therefore, the main cause of pulmonary oedema is not dilution but elevation of capillary pressure by excess fluids [1, 20]. This is just as likely to happen with colloids, indeed, at equal rates of infusion, more so because of the greater retention within the circulation. While colloids imitate the effect of plasma proteins they do not replace them because their effects are short lived and unlike albumin, their charge confers little ability to hold additional sodium in circulation and thus further boost circulating volume [21].

The advantage of colloids, therefore, is that they boost circulating volume, though not as well as albumin, and enable crystalloids to be held in circulation rather than inappropriately boosting interstitial fluid. They are not necessarily safer than crystalloids but almost certainly more effective than the use of crystalloids alone.

Cellular aspects

The cellular effects of shock remain the least understood and thus the most intractable aspects. Partly they result from the factors already considered, i.e. redistribution of blood flow, progressive ischaemia, deterioration of plasma composition, etc. Substantially, however, they are also part of a more generalized metabolic response to trauma which can be triggered by any injury of sufficient severity and which often, therefore, accompanies shock [1, 22–24].

Among the features of this response are initial impairment of metabolism (ebb phase) with mobilization of glucose but impaired utilization. Body temperature falls, partly as a result of a regulated resetting of 'set-point' which may improve survival but also because the metabolic changes interfere with the ability to increase heat production in response to cooling. It is therefore desirable to limit heat loss although actual warming is counterproductive since it may cause sufficient vasodilation to undermine the preservation of adequate arterial pressure. Later in the aftermath of trauma there is acceleration of metabolic rate, mobilization of stores (glycogen, fat, protein) and conversion to fuels (glucose, fatty acids, amino acids); since glycogen stores are relatively slender there is a risk of hypoglycaemia which may contribute to the terminal effects of shock. Full development of 'flow phase' outlasts shock, depends on circulatory recovery and may elevate body temperature without infection.

The hormonal factors mediating these metabolic responses to trauma are not well understood, partly because so many hormones with effects on metabolism are found in higher concentration either as a result of increased secretion or reduced breakdown [1, 22].

Among these are the corticosteroids but the endogenous levels never approach the levels attained by the 'pharmacological doses' advocated for the treatment of shock. Catecholamines (e.g. adrenaline) also increase and thus contribute to the metabolic as well as the circulatory effects of shock. They promote the hyperglycaemia, not only by mobilizing glucose but by suppressing insulin [22]. Cells also become insulin-resistant, partly as a result of membrane damage [24].

The early hyperglycaemia may have some beneficial effect in drawing fluid from cells and promoting transfer not only of interstitial fluid but its accompanying protein back to plasma [1]. Although the concentration of protein in interstitial fluid is much less than plasma, the volume is so much larger that interstitial fluid can provide a significant reserve. Interest in this hyperglycaemia and its osmotic effects has led to a quite separate area of research on highly concentrated fluids in the treatment of shock [2]. They act by causing reflex improvements in cardiovascular function unrelated to volume replacement. Like research on direct metabolic intervention with substances such as Mg-ATP, this work remains experimental [1]. Nevertheless, it is part of a growing indication that the next major step forward in the treatment of shock will be the ability to understand and correct the cellular and metabolic changes, rather than further refinements in managing the cardiovascular problem. Such advances are crucial because eventually in advanced shock, restoration of circulation is unable to reverse the metabolic changes, i.e. by current means the shock is truly irreversible [24].

Summary: major adverse effects of shock

Vascular changes
1 Changes in vascular tone (especially excess vasoconstriction).
2 Changes in vascular permeability (increased).

Changes in blood
1 Reduced volume.
2 Increased viscosity.
3 Excessive/impaired tendency to clot.

Cardiac function
Depressed: deterioration of plasma composition; MDF.

Deterioration of plasma composition
1 Increased K^+.
2 Increased H^+.
3 (Eventually) hypoglycaemia.

Changes in cell metabolism:
Numerous and, as yet, almost beyond specific therapy.

Classification of shock

So far the discussion of shock has treated it as a single condition whereas several forms can be distinguished [1]. The most important, and the model for the general features, is *hypovolaemic shock* (often caused by trauma, sometimes by haemorrhage so that traumatic or haemorrhagic shock are almost synonymous).

Vasogenic or neurogenic shock begins differently, with inappropriate vascular tone as the initiating cause, rather than circulating volume or cardiac output. Inappropriate vasodilatation can be the primary factor (e.g. after spinal injury or anaesthesia) though with compensatory vasoconstriction the subsequent stages converge on a similar 'final common path'. Inappropriate vasoconstriction resulting from pain or visceral traction can also contribute to neurogenic shock.

Cardiogenic shock is initiated by reduced cardiac output following myocardial failure. Both these forms of shock are much less common in animals. *Anaphylactic shock* is triggered by an antigen–antibody interaction which leads to high concentration of histamine and other mediators in circulation. These may initially cause peripheral pooling of blood or peripheral vasoconstriction but subsequently, despite its distinctive features, the final common path has much in common with hypovolaemic shock. Indeed, shock generally involves localized accumulations of histamine without the marked systemic increase. Prostaglandins also increase during shock but it remains uncertain whether their predominant effects are harmful or beneficial (see below).

Endotoxic shock is important in animals, initiated by the breakdown products of dead or dying bacteria. The emphasis is on inappropriate vascular tone rather than hypovolaemia [1, 25]. There is venous pooling leading to diminished cardiac output. There may also be localized overperfusion of infected tissue and changes in capillary permeability. The response, however, is vasoconstriction so that the 'final common path' again resembles traumatic shock. Although the formation of endotoxin can be increased by bactericidal drugs [26−28], there are no reports of adverse effects resulting from their use in clinical cases of shock; the paramount objective is to prevent further proliferation or spread of bacteria.

Septic shock involves the additional presence of bacteria in circulation [3, 29, 30]; there may be sufficient regional over-perfusion to initially increase cardiac output, despite the under-perfusion of most tissues. Unlike hypovolaemic shock, endotoxin shock tends to depress gluconeogenesis and, therefore, leads to earlier development of hypo-glycaemia as well as poorer utilization of lactate [31].

Monitoring of shock

The main objective in monitoring of a patient in shock is to recognize and treat any deficiencies in tissue perfusion as soon as they develop.

Many techniques are available, some simple, others more sophisticated, but even with minimal equipment valuable information can be gained.

Essential monitoring

Minimal cardio-circulatory monitoring requires the recording of pulse rate and rhythm. Changes in pulse rate and volume are frequently present in shock and provide a useful check of how the animal is responding to therapy. Palpation of peripheral pulses will also indicate the state of peripheral perfusion and whether there is intense vaso-constriction. The patient in shock has a rapid, weak and thready pulse.

Respiration should also be monitored. Hypovolaemic animals frequently hyperventilate and a return to a more normal respiratory pattern is therefore a favourable sign. Regular auscultation of the chest will also enable early detection of fluid rales or increased harshness of respiratory sounds which might indicate the development of pulmonary oedema.

Ventilometry: ventilation rates alone give little information on the adequacy of ventilation, although a change in rate often gives a sign that all is not well. Ideally, tidal volume is measured but some estimate at least may be made by looking at the chest wall movement.

Temperature: animals in shock have labile body temperatures and the vasoconstriction produced in response to hypovolaemia causes the temperature of peripheral tissue to fall so that the gradient between the core temperature and the periphery widens (Table 4.1). Thus the temperature difference between the toes and oesophageal or rectal temperature is a useful guide to peripheral perfusion. Thermister probes are ideal for measuring both core and peripheral temperatures (Fig. 4.4). Although rectal temperature is a less satisfactory approximation of core temperature than measurements of oesophageal temperature, it is adequate for clinical use. The normal gradient is usually no more than 3–4°C but widens to more than 10–12°C in hypovolaemic shock. Toe web temperature falls due to peripheral vasoconstriction and skin temperature approaches ambient. An animal in shock, *whatever the primary cause,* becomes hypothermic, i.e. its core temperature falls.

Central venous pressure monitoring (CVP) is easily measured [32] (Chapter 5) and can be a guide to right ventricular function and the degree of hypovolaemia present since it represents the balance between venous return and cardiac output. In an animal with inadequate circulation, a CVP above the normal range for the species is likely to

Table 4.1 Toe web–rectal temperature gradient in normal and hypovolaemic dogs under anaesthesia

Toe web temperature (°C)	Rectal temperature (°C)	Difference (°C)
Normal dogs		
32.6	37.0	4.4
33.2	36.8	3.6
34.0	36.8	2.8
35.0	38.6	3.6
Hypovolaemic dogs		
28.0	36.8	8.8
30.0	36.0	6.0
25.0	36.0	11.0
26.0	35.0	9.0

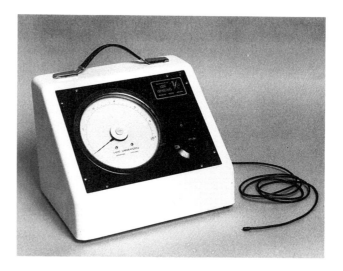

Fig. 4.4 Equipment for the measurement of core−peripheral temperature gradient.

be due to cardiac failure, while a low CVP is likely to be due to hypovolaemia. If the CVP value is equivocal the possibility that the circulatory failure may be due to hypovolaemia may be tested by a fluid challenge in which 1 ml/kg of colloid solution is transfused over a 2 minute period. If the vascular system is relatively empty there will be a small transient increase in the CVP; vascular congestion or cardiac failure will result in a larger, more prolonged increase in the CVP.

Isolated measurements are of little value because an animal may have a normal or even elevated CVP despite being hypovolaemic in the presence of hypoxia, hypercapnia, or chronic pulmonary fibrosis associated with pulmonary hypertension. In addition, the infusion of vasoactive drugs (e.g. adrenaline, isoprenaline for inotropic support) will result in vasoconstriction of the systemic veins and raise the CVP even in the presence of severe hypovolaemia. In septic shock or endotoxaemia arteriolar vasodilatation occurs so that arterial pressure is transmitted more directly to the central veins, thus maintaining a high CVP even if the blood volume is low. In tricuspid valvular incompetence the right ventricular pressure will be transmitted to the CVP manometer through the incompetent valve.

In any of these conditions the CVP will be high even when hypovolaemia is present yet the presence of circulatory failure will be shown by a fast pulse rate, cold extremities and arterial hypotension. Despite the raised CVP there may still be hypovolaemia since the left ventricular filling pressure may be inadequate. Ideally, in all these cases the left ventricular filling pressure should be determined by measurement of the pulmonary artery wedge pressure (PAWP) or preferably pulmonary artery diastolic pressure (if practicable). If there are signs of circulatory failure and the PAWP is low, then transfusion is indicated, in spite of the high CVP, until the PAWP is increased sufficiently to give adequate filling of the left ventricle. Conversely, CVP may still be slightly low when organ perfusion as judged by other parameters (urine output, core–periphery temperature gradient) is acceptable. It must be remembered that some normal animals have a low CVP and it is quite futile to try to raise the CVP in an animal which has pink mucous membranes, warm extremities and a good urine production, for the excess fluid infused will simply pass out as urine.

Overall, CVP is probably of less value than other parameters in judging whether enough fluid has been given. In human medicine, much more weight is placed on the CVP response to fluid challenge. If the CVP rises and stays high after a rapid fluid challenge, this is taken as an indication that the infusion rate should be considerably slowed whereas if the CVP falls fairly quickly, then this usually indicates that more fluids can be infused safely. CVP tends to rise more rapidly, i.e. prematurely, in acidosis [33].

Urine output is the single most useful measurement that can be made. Urine production is sensitive to glomerular filtration rate and therefore to renal perfusion and, indirectly, to blood pressure. A reduced rate of urine production therefore indicates severe hypovolaemia/hypotension, while a return of production is a good prognostic sign. It is important to realize that low urine output can also result from acute renal failure (Chapter 10).

Urine production is best measured by inserting a urinary catheter. After emptying the bladder, urine is collected and measured hourly either by continuous or intermittent drainage. In more active animals, the catheter may need to be taped or sutured in place.

Normal urine production is conventionally estimated to be around 1–1.5 ml/kg/hour; a flow of less than 0.5 ml/kg/hour may be considered to constitute oliguria.

Capillary refill time (CRT): after digital pressure on a mucous membrane, the capillaries momentarily blanch. Normally they refill immediately (<1 second) but in shock, refilling takes longer because of arteriolar vasoconstriction (CRT >3 seconds). When venous pressure is elevated by heart failure, CRT may be normal even in the presence of shock. Poor capillary refill must not be disregarded, but normal CRT does not guarantee adequate perfusion. It can be especially misleading in anaesthetized animals.

Additional monitoring

1 Blood pressure, and pulmonary artery wedge pressure measurements.
2 Blood gases, hydrogen ion status, Pao_2.
3 Biochemical changes (blood sugar, lactate).
4 ECG.

Blood pressure

Arterial blood pressure tends to fall in advanced shock and hypotension seems to be one of the most reliable adverse prognostic indicators in colic in the horse [34]. More sophisticated and much less essential information may be obtained by pulmonary wedge pressure measurements and cardiac output determinations. Flow directed balloon catheters are used to gauge pulmonary wedge pressure as an index of left ventricular function. Cardiac output may be determined using these catheters and a thermal dilution technique.

Blood gases

The most accurate way of determining the adequacy of alveolar ventilation is to measure arterial CO_2 and O_2 levels. In shock, hyperventilation often leads to decreased levels of CO_2 initially while arterial oxygen tensions are maintained within the normal range. Venous O_2 tensions tend to fall as tissues extract their oxygen from the increasingly sluggish blood flow; very low venous Po_2 levels can indicate severe shock.

At the same time as measuring blood gases, the blood gas machine will measure pH and, by calculation, determine the bicarbonate concentration in the blood and the base deficit. Severe shock tends to produce a metabolic acidosis with a base deficit of around 10–15 mmol/l. Table 4.2 illustrates this, with blood gas measurements made in horses suffering severe colic as a result of gastrointestinal obstruction/ischaemia (Chapter 12). Fortunately, simple measurements of total CO_2 (TCO_2) provide useful information regarding blood bicarbonate and, therefore, the severity of metabolic acidosis.

Biochemical and haematological changes

Although lactic acidosis tends to develop in shock, its severity does not appear to provide a reliable prognostic guide, except in extremes [34]. A direct relationship between blood lactate and mortality has been claimed by many workers but others found it of less direct clinical usefulness than, for example, measurement of anion gap [35, 36]. Cowan and his colleagues [37] carried out an interesting prospective study, comparing the prognostic value of lactate concentration and haemodynamic changes in patients with septic shock. Although serial lactate measurements were more useful than single estimations, they were much less reliable than simple haemodynamic variables like urine output, core–peripheral temperature gradients and changes in arterial blood pressure.

Haematology: initially the haematocrit will be unchanged in shock, unless the hypovolaemia is due to dehydration in which case it rises. Following haemorrhage, the main value in monitoring the

Table 4.2 Blood gas measurements in horses with colic

Animal	Problem	pH	P_{CO_2}	P_{O_2}	[HCO_3^-]	Base deficit
			Jugular venous blood			
Shire foal (M)	8 ft gangrenous intestine resected (L)	7.231	46.0	44.4	19.3	8.3
TB (M)	Torsion root of mesentery (D)	7.042	66.2	49.8	15.4	16.4
TB (F)	Gangrenous SI (D)	7.158	40.5	65.0	14.3	14.1
TB 3 year (MN)	Caecal infarction (L)	7.307	52.9	54.8	26.4	0.6
2 year (MN)	Intussusception (L)	7.262	46.7	67.6	21.0	6.1
13 year (MN)	Lipoma on stalk, strangulating SI, peritonitis (D)	7.060	37.8	53.9	10.8	19.4

D = died; F = female; L = lived; M = male; MN = neutered male/gelding; SI = small intestine; TB = thoroughbred.

haematocrit is to help decide when a whole blood transfusion becomes indicated, i.e. PCV is below 20 and falling. In advanced shock
elevated PCV reflects fluid loss from leaky capillaries and warns of
high viscosity as an added impediment to oxygen delivery.

Blood glucose: blood glucose levels rise initially following trauma, due
to the effect of sympathetic system activation and generally, the
higher the level, the poorer is the prognosis; ultimately hypoglycaemia
supervenes and requires treatment.

ECG

The ECG may change following severe haemorrhage. Reduction in
ventricular volume associated with hypovolaemia will cause a decrease
in the amplitude of the R-wave in the QRS complex (ventricular
depolarization) of the ECG. Severe myocardial hypoxia or severe
acidosis will also result in ectopic ventricular beats.

Therapeutic implications

The pathophysiological and pharmacological factors already discussed
lead to the following conclusions:
1 Urgent replacement of circulating volume with a fluid of broadly
plasma-like composition is an essential priority (see also Chapter 3).
2 Unless haemorrhage is severe, blood is not needed and may be
contraindicated (see also Chapter 8).
3 Despite their advantages, colloids are not necessarily safer (with
regard to pulmonary oedema) and, at least with dextrans, there is
some risk of side effects, notably in horses (see also Chapter 3).
4 There is substantial justification for the use of antibiotics.
5 Antihistamines, if they are to be beneficial, must be used very
early.
6 Systemic vasoconstrictors are contraindicated except for adrenaline
in anaphylactic shock.
7 Vasodilators (α-blockers) may be beneficial but only if volume
replacement is well under way.

The theoretical and experimental merits of numerous drugs have
failed to live up to expectation in clinical use [1, 2]. Nevertheless,
there is substantial reason to expect progress with the use of anti-
endorphin drugs such as naloxone, and also to anticipate the increasing

use of non-steroidal anti-inflammatory agents. Dopamine appears to have very useful cardiovascular effects but is somewhat inconvenient (sustained infusion). Corticosteroids are probably a useful adjunct to fluid therapy provided they are used early and in massive doses; they are unlikely to do harm (see below).

In the longer term, the main advances seem likely to concern:

1 Prevention of reticuloendothelial depression.

2 Correction of cellular metabolic disturbances.

3 Development of a convenient, safe and inexpensive blood substitute.

Treatment of shock

Hypovolaemic shock

Restoration of circulating volume

The most important feature of hypovolaemic shock is the reduction in the circulating blood volume, which occurs due to either external or occult losses of blood, plasma or body fluids.

The first line of treatment must therefore be the replacement of this *'lost fluid'*. The exact choice of replacement fluid depends to a great extent on the type of loss which has been incurred, but in the last few years a slight change of emphasis has occurred. Previously, it was considered important to replace any blood loss 'in kind' with losses being predicted from clinical signs. Nowadays it is generally accepted that one cannot be dogmatic about the amount of fluid which needs to be given and indeed, the best guide to the adequacy of replacement is the animal's response to treatment.

The paramount importance of replacing blood which is lost with an equivalent volume of whole blood has also been questioned. It is now generally agreed that a haemoglobin level of about 10 g/dl and a PCV of around 30−35% are optimum for blood flow to tissues as the blood's viscosity is minimized at this concentration. While there can be no doubt that severe depletion of the intravascular fluid due to haemorrhage is best treated by the transfusion of stored blood or red cells, these commodities are likely always to be in short supply in veterinary practice. Even when blood is needed, it is usually supplemented with a greater volume of electrolyte or colloidal solution [39]. Thus, under most circumstances the veterinarian is faced with the decision as to whether colloids or crystalloids should be used and in what quantities.

The arguments over the choice of either colloidal or crystalloid solutions for the resuscitation of animals in shock continue, based on both experimental and clinical investigations. There is no doubt that excessive use of lactated Ringer's solution was a major cause of respiratory difficulties in patients in Vietnam and over-transfusion of dogs with crystalloid solutions will produce pulmonary oedema [40]. However, provided the animal has normal renal and cardiovascular function, the adverse effects of over-transfusion are generally short lived. Theoretically, overload with a colloid solution is potentially more dangerous as the colloids remain in the circulation for longer, but provided overload is avoided, colloids confer decided advantages in treating hypovolaemia [41]. Frequently a combination of both is required, to avoid excess colloid and also on the grounds of cost.

When colloid solutions are not available, crystalloids alone may be used on the basis that they do repair ECF volume. The disadvantage of infusing crystalloids is that they are not confined within the vascular bed but equilibrate with the whole of the extracellular fluid (Chapter 3). Thus 75% of the infused fluid enters the interstitial space whether or not this space needs replenishment, whereas the aim is to correct plasma deficits implied by observations such as changes in pulse rate, peripheral temperature, arterial pressure and urine output. Any excess in interstitial fluid is not clinically recognizable unless it is gross — when peripheral oedema may be observable. Colloids will correct intravascular volume deficits more rapidly than crystalloids and more efficiently; less fluid is required, plasma osmotic pressure is not reduced so peripheral oedema is avoided and tissue oxygen exchange is not impaired.

No generally available intravenous solution has oxygen-carrying capacity although fluorocarbon solutions have been used for this purpose and may soon be more freely available. The problems in obtaining safe blood for human transfusion have intensified the search for safe, convenient blood substitutes, able to function at atmospheric oxygen tensions. Once they are developed, and become cost effective, they will almost certainly be suitable for veterinary use. For the present, however, when losses of blood become critical, whole blood infusion becomes essential.

Initially, in resuscitation, the type of fluid used is of less importance than swift establishment of a rapid infusion. Only when the intravenous line has been placed and fluids are going in fast, should one stop to reconsider if one has made the ideal choice. Up to 3 ml/kg/ minute may be infused in the first minutes, slowing to 1−1.5 ml/kg/ minute for the next half hour or so until the animal's condition starts to improve. Needless to say, these high flow rates are achieved only by using large gauge needles or catheters placed in reasonably sized veins, or by setting up several lines in smaller veins.

Assessment of the adequacy of treatment is based almost entirely on the animal's clinical response and the means of assessing this has already been discussed. Monitoring is literally vital in shock; the more thoroughly it can be done, the better the likelihood of successful treatment.

Other measures

In most cases, restoration of the circulating blood volume is all that is required. However, it may occasionally be necessary to use other measures to improve peripheral blood flow.

1 *Dextrans.* Since blood viscosity increases in shock, the infusion of a low molecular weight dextran (40) may be indicated, although usually fluid replacement therapy by virtue of causing a degree of haemodilution is all that is required.

2 The use of *inotropic* agents such as dopamine or dobutamine can be beneficial especially if myocardial function is deteriorating. Dopamine has the added advantage of improving renal blood flow by virtue of stimulating renal dopaminergic receptors and is a relatively safe drug. Dobutamine on the other hand, is a pure β_1 agonist which seems to work principally by improving stroke volume rather than heart rate. The other β agonist, isoprenaline, also improves cardiac output but causes a marked tachycardia and is therefore more likely to cause dysrhythmias than the other drugs mentioned.

3 If tissue perfusion does not improve despite adequate fluid replacement therapy, *α-adrenergic blockage* may be indicated. Specific vasodilators such as phenoxybenzamine (long-lasting, irreversible), or thymoxamine (shorter-acting) or phentolamine are often used in humans but acepromazine or chlorpromazine are alternatives. It cannot be over-emphasized that the use of these drugs in hypovolaemic animals must be avoided as the generalized vasodilation which they induce can cause a disastrous fall in venous return. The results of their use are monitored principally by measuring the core–skin temperature (see above).

Cardiogenic shock

Myocardial infarction is rare in animals but cardiac decompensation may occur in dogs with chronic valvular disease. Cardiac performance may also be severely impaired if there is a cardiac tamponade, tension pneumothorax or obstruction of the vena cava. The release of myocardial depressant factor (MDF) from the ischaemic pancreas in circulatory shock also means that myocardial depression is a frequent complicating factor in all types of shock. Acute cardiac failure may also develop if the chordae tendinae rupture.

The most severe manifestation of cardiac failure, especially with left heart disease, is pulmonary oedema. This is best managed by:
1 Providing an increased inspired oxygen concentration.
2 Giving diuretics. Frusemide at a dose rate of up to 10 mg/kg should be given intravenously. This dose may be repeated in 2–3 hours if necessary.
3 If diuretics do not cause an improvement in the animal's condition within a few hours, then cardiac glycoside therapy may be tried. Digitalis is extremely toxic in the hypovolaemic, hypoxic animal and its use is therefore best avoided in the acute stages of cardiogenic shock. Severe arrhythmias can be easily provoked in the hypoxic myocardium and ECG monitoring is considered essential so that should dysrhythmias occur, they can be promptly treated.
4 Reduce the 'afterload' on the heart by reducing peripheral vascular resistance, i.e. use vasodilators, either α-adrenergic antagonists such as thymoxamine, phentolamine or phenoxybenzamine (all 1 mg/kg) or directly acting vasodilators.

Septic shock

Volume replacement

Many animals which develop signs of septicaemia may have been hypovolaemic and will need large volumes of fluids; however, others clearly need fluids despite having no obvious fluid loss. *This is the main feature of the 'leaky capillary problem' in septic shock.* Because of capillary endothelial damage, pulmonary capillary leak and pulmonary oedema is very common in septicaemic shock and the margin for error between over-transfusion and inadequate volume replacement is much narrower. Because of this leakiness of capillaries, on balance, it may be safer to use colloids rather than large volumes of crystalloids in septicaemic shock.

Control infection

Naturally, the source of infection should be dealt with at the earliest opportunity. In addition, antibiotics should be used. Ideally, the choice of antibiotic should be dictated by bacteriological findings, but this is not often possible, and treatment has to begin well before laboratory results are to hand. A balanced broad spectrum combination which should include drugs active against Gram-negative organisms should be continued for at least 5 days.

In view of the susceptibility of dogs in shock (whatever the cause) to succumb to intestinal mucosal ischaemia and septicaemia, antibiotic therapy is always essential in this species. Treatment should be intravenous, using high doses of the drugs repeated at least 8-hourly.

Support organ function

Septicaemia often results in the development of hyponatraemia as cell damage occurs and the sodium pump fails causing the so-called sick cell syndrome. As a consequence, sodium and water accumulate intracellularly and potassium leaks out into the extracellular fluid. The diagnosis of this syndrome is difficult but is made by comparing measured plasma osmolality with that calculated from electrolyte levels in the plasma [42]. A large discrepancy indicates the presence of unmeasured ions and is suggestive of sick cell syndrome. Treatment is difficult but an insulin and glucose infusion should help to stimulate the sodium pump which will then move sodium out of cells, and return potassium to them from ECF.

General measures

The most elementary step is to treat the cause, as far as possible, e.g. arrest continuing haemorrhage and to maximize oxygen delivery, i.e. check the airway and provide respiratory support if need be.

Treating metabolic acidosis

Once shock becomes established, impaired tissue perfusion soon leads to the development of a metabolic acidosis. Sodium bicarbonate will therefore be required to correct this if myocardial function and blood viscosity is not to be adversely affected. If the base deficit can be measured (see above), then the amount of additional bicarbonate required can be titrated accurately. Otherwise 2.5 mmol/kg may be given fairly safely. This sort of amount will help a moderate to severe acidosis without producing a serious alkalosis, should the animal not have a base deficit. Whether or not additional bicarbonate is used, volume replacement with solutions lacking bicarbonate or a precursor should be avoided.

Improving the inspired oxygen concentration (FIO_2)

This is beneficial provided that the advantages of improving oxygen flux are not outweighed by an increased oxygen consumption rate should the animal struggle and not tolerate the application of a mask. Smaller animals can be successfully treated in an improvised oxygen tent or incubator. Oxygen by nasal catheter, provided it is first warmed and humidified, is often surprisingly well tolerated by large animals.

Body heat should be conserved

Body temperature usually falls in shock, especially once the animal loses its thermoregulatory ability. Hypothermia should be avoided by preventing heat loss and nursing the animal in a warm environment (at least 25°C if possible). Direct application of heat should be avoided as this may not only provoke peripheral vasodilation but may also cause skin burns (and sloughs) if the animal is so ill that it is unable to move. All intravenous fluids should be warmed to 37−40°C before administration in order to avoid incurring a thermal debt. Polystyrene containers or polystyrene chips provide useful insulation.

Antibiotics

The justification for using antibiotics in shocked animals is not just the presence of contaminated wounds but the risk of invasion by bacteria from the gut [1]. Like so many aspects of the adjunctive therapy of shock, we are sadly short of definitive trials and final decisions must rest to a considerable degree on individual judgement and experience. There is certainly little evidence of the clinical use of antibiotics exacerbating any form of shock.

Other measures which are often used in treating shock are not specific to the treatment of hypovolaemic shock but are used when the initial resuscitation has been delayed and the patient has entered the second phase which is characterized by tissue damage and serious metabolic consequences common to other sorts of shock (see above). Suffice to say that in uncomplicated hypovolaemic shock, there is no clear need for corticosteroids or any of the other more controversial measures sometimes advocated. Nevertheless, since shock is potentially lethal, there is justification for a variety of measures which may be beneficial.

The need for the treatments discussed so far is fairly widely accepted. A number of other approaches are now discussed which are 'controversial' in the sense that either they are widely used but not rigorously proven or they are relatively new and time is still needed to assess their real value.

Controversial treatment measures

Corticosteroids

The use of glucocorticoids in the treatment of shock is surrounded by controversy and a voluminous amount of published work. Despite numerous reports either for or against their use, objective, controlled trials are conspicuously absent [1].

Corticosteroids have a wide spectrum of activity against an astonishing range of the harmful effects of shock [1]. There is a strong body of clinical opinion that they are beneficial in high doses, especially against endotoxin or septic shock [43]. Unfortunately, there has been great difficulty in providing convincing demonstrations of these potential virtues in well designed clinical trials [1]. There is, however, little likelihood of harm when appropriately used and it is probable that they are a useful adjunct to fluid therapy, provided they are used early [1, 2]. A possible exception is in horses and ponies, where potentially adverse effects have been found such as delayed healing, risk of infection and laminitis [44].

When used in massive doses (30 mg/kg methylprednisolone; 10 mg/kg dexamethasone), corticosteroids act pharmacologically to cause vasodilatation, improved cardiac output and tissue perfusion. Pulmonary oedema is less likely as lysosomal and other cell membranes are stabilized. Pretreatment with steroids is certainly protective against endotoxin shock. The controversy arises over whether steroids are equally effective when given after the onset of shock, since pretreatment is highly unlikely to be possible in clinical cases.

There have been few attempts at evaluating steroids in dogs; one study showed a beneficial effect only when given within 15 minutes of endotoxin challenge and then only if combined with antibiotics. Another demonstrated an increased survival rate only if given early and in combination with large volumes of fluids. In humans the conclusion is still that while prolongation of life for 24 hours may be improved, full recovery rates are unaltered.

All the positive evidence, such as there is, refers to the effectiveness of steroids in endotoxin and septic shock; their value in hypovolaemic shock is even more dubious. However, despite this, we can at least say that their use is not deleterious, and since there is a strong body of clinical opinion that they may be beneficial, they are often used in treating shock. It is important to remember that if they are used, they should be considered to be additional measures and not as an alternative to fluid therapy. A recent and disturbing development is that steroids are now regarded as being contraindicated in humans with endotoxic/septic shock — the one circumstance in which any reasonable clinical trial data supported their use [2].

The pulmonary complications of shock — so-called 'shock lung' are undoubtedly responsible for the ultimate death of many animals following major trauma. The implication of activation of the complement cascade and the damage to pulmonary capillaries by microaggregates (and the kinins they release) in the generation of 'shock lung' makes the administration of large doses of steroids a sensible measure in these cases.

Non-steroidal anti-inflammatory drugs

Many workers have shown that prostaglandins may mediate some effects of shock especially endotoxin shock and antagonists such as flunixin have been demonstrated to be partially protective against

endotoxic shock in dogs and horses [2, 44]. Nevertheless, some prostaglandin effects are beneficial in shock, e.g. stabilization of lysosomes
and reduced production of MDF [1].

Antihistamines

Pretreatment with antihistamines such as promethazine has been
demonstrated to be effective in preventing the onset of shock [1] but
delay in administration beyond 30 minutes renders this drug ineffec-
tive. This need for pretreatment clearly limits the clinical usefulness of
this line of treatment.

Heparin

In view of the predilection for the formation of micro-aggregates in
poorly perfused capillaries in shock, some workers recommend the
administration of heparin in order to prevent the development of
disseminated intravascular coagulation. In practice it would seem
more prudent to avoid this drug in the absence of specialist laboratory facilities. Treatment of animals which have recently suffered
major trauma or surgery with heparin is fraught with the risk of
haemorrhage.

Naloxone

The endogenous opiate β-endorphin is known to be released from the
pituitary during shock states and may well contribute to the hypotension produced in both haemorrhagic and endotoxin shock.
Naloxone has been shown to reverse this hypotension and may well
be efficacious in treating septic shock if given in large enough doses
(10 mg/kg). Its use raises questions, however, concerning possible
restoration of pain sensitivity which is usually reduced in shock.

Hypertonic saline

There are promising indications that the use of small volumes of
hypertonic saline may prove beneficial in the treatment of shock
[1, 2]. The mechanisms reflect improved cardiopulmonary function,
partly reflex mediated, together with improved peripheral perfusion.
The approach is quite distinct from fluid therapy, i.e. volume replace-

ment, and is simple since it uses small volumes. For the moment, however, its value remains a matter of experimental investigation and it cannot yet be regarded as established therapy.

Conclusion

'Irreversible shock' is a familiar term but it means no more than irreversible within the limits set by:

1 The general clinical context: how satisfactory a recovery is in prospect, if shock is survived and whether there are economic or humanitarian constraints on how much effort and materials should be invested.

2 The facilities and assistance available.

3 The severity or duration of the individual case.

Of course some cases would be irreversible in any circumstances; current knowledge remains insufficient to match every need. But there is no measurement or sign which marks the boundary between reversible and irreversible shock so precisely as to define when a case is not worth treating. In the interests of the patient any case of shock must be regarded as potentially reversible, at least initially.

We have made some distinction between measures which are reasonably routine and others which are more controversial; even this depends on the viewpoint of different clinicians. The use of 'controversial' measures, provided they have no adverse effect, will ultimately make them routine even before or without the availability of definitive clinical trials. Shock is a rapidly progressive and lethal condition; the individual patient cannot afford the luxury of waiting for p to equal 0.001 before taking advantage of any measure which has a strong basis for a likely beneficial effect, and little reason or evidence to indicate that its use would be detrimental.

The approach to shock continuously demands evaluation and reassessment, not only of the individual case but the overall strategies. So long as wars and major accidents continue, research efforts will remain intense and will necessitate frequent revision; routines will be modified accordingly. But the approach to the individual case will always need to be fast and decisive. Hesitation merely allows time for the vicious cycles to multiply and for the problems to progress from the circulatory changes which we understand best to the cellular disturbances which remain beyond our understanding and our therapy.

References

1 Michell, A.R. (1985) What is shock? *Journal of Small Animal Practice* **26**, 719–38.
2 Michell, A.R. (1989) Shock in companion animals. In: *Veterinary Annual*, Vol. 29. Grunsell, C.S.G. & Hill, F.W.G. (eds). Butterworth, London.
3 Janssen, H.F. & Barnes, C.D. (1985) *Circulatory Shock: Basic and Clinical Implications*, 1–22. Academic Prees, London.
4 Michell, A.R. (1979) Fluid therapy: some specific applications to medical conditions in small animals. *Veterinary Record* **104**, 572–5.
5 Hunt, T.K., Rabkin, J. & Van Smitten, K. (1986) Effect of edema and anemia on wound healing and infection. In: *Albumin and the Systemic Circulation*, 101–13. Blauhut, B. & Lundsgaard-Hansen, P. (eds). Karger, Basel.
6 Michell, A.R. (1983) Understanding fluid therapy. *Irish Veterinary Journal* **37**, 94–103.
7 Brasmer, T.H. (1984) *The Acutely Traumatised Small Animal Patient*, 97–113. W.B. Saunders, Philadelphia.
8 Bennett, B. & Towler, H.M.A. (1985) Haemostatic response to trauma. *British Medical Bulletin* **41**, 274–80.
9 Longnecker, D.E. (1983) Anaesthesia. In: *Handbook of Shock and Trauma*, Vol. 1, 449–59. Altura, B.M., Lefer, A.M. & Schumer, W. (eds). Raven, New York.
10 Haglund, U. (1983) Shock toxins. *British Medical Bulletin* **41**, 377–92.
11 Haskins, S.C. (1983) Shock. In: *Current Veterinary Therapy VIII*, 2–27. Kirk, R.W. (ed). Saunders, Philadelphia.
12 Loegering, D.J. (1981) Presence of a reticuloendothelial depressing substance in portal vein blood following intestinal ischaemia and thermal injury. *Advances in Shock Research* **5**, 67–73.
13 Cohen, J.J. & Kassirer, J.P. (1982) Metabolic acidosis. *Acid–Base*, 121–226. Little Brown, Boston.
14 Kopple, J.D. & Blumenkrantz, M.J. (1980) In: *Clinical Disorders of Fluid and Electrolyte Metabolism*, 472–6. Maxwell, M.H. & Kleeman, C.R. (eds). McGraw Hill, New York.
15 Relman, A.S. (1978) Lactic acidosis. In: *Acid–Base and Potassium Homeostasis*, 65–101. Brenner, B.M. & Stein, J.H. (eds). Churchill Livingstone, New York.
16 Hartsfield, S.M., Thurman, J.C. & Benson, G.J. (1981) Sodium bicarbonate and bicarbonate precursors for treatment of metabolic acidosis. *Journal of the American Veterinary Medical Association* **179**, 914–6.
17 Ballard, F.J. (1972) Supply and utilisation of acetate in mammals. *American Journal of Clinical Nutrition* **25**, 773–9.
18 Michell, A.R. (1988) Drips, drinks and drenches; what matters in fluid therapy? *Irish Veterinary Journal* **42**, 17–22.
19 Lutz, H. & Georgieff, M. (1986) In: *Albumin and the Systemic Circulation*, 145–54. Blauhut, B. & Lundgaard-Hansen, P. (eds). Karger, Basel.
20 Demling, R.H. (1986) In: *Albumin and the Systemic Circulation*, 36–63. Blauhut, B. & Lundgaard-Hansen, P. (eds). Karger, Basel.
21 Veech, R.L. (1986) The toxic impact of parenteral solutions on the metabolism of cells. *American Journal of Clinical Nutrition*, **44**, 519–51.
22 Aulick, L.H. & Wilmore, D.W. (1983) Hypermetabolism in trauma. In: *Mammalian Thermogenesis*, 259–303. Girardier, L. & Stock, M.J. (eds). Chapman & Hall, London.
23 Michell, A.R. (1974) The metabolic consequences of trauma. *Journal of Small Animal Practice* **15**, 279–91.
24 Heath, D.F. (1985) Subcellular aspects of the response to trauma. *British Medical Bulletin* **41**, 240–5.

25 Jennings, P.B., Whitten, N.J. & Sleeman, H.K. (1981) The diagnosis and treatment of shock in the critical care patient. In: *Veterinary Critical Care*, 485–523. Settler, F.D., Knowles, R.P. & Whittick, W.G. (eds). Lea & Febiger, Philadelphia.

26 Shenep, J.L. & Mogan, K.A. (1984) Kinetics of endotoxin release during antibiotic therapy for experimental gram-negative bacterial sepsis. *Journal of Infectious Diseases* **150**, 380–8.

27 Jacobson, M.A. & Young, L.S. (1985) Gram-negative shock: approaches to treatment. *Journal of the Royal College of Physicians, London* **19**, 214–7.

28 McAnulty, J.F. (1983) Septic shock in the dog: A review. *Journal of American Animal Hospital Association* **19**, 827–35.

29 Hardie, E.M. & Rawlings, C.A. (1983) Septic shock. *Compendium of Continuing Education for the Practising Veterinarian* **5**, 369–77; 483–93.

30 Schumer, W. (1984) Subcellular response to septic shock. In: *Shock and Related Problems*, 61–9. Shires, G.T. (ed). Churchill Livingstone, London.

31 Phillips, R.W. & Case, G.L. (1980) Altered metabolism, acute shock and therapeutic response in a calf with severe coronavirus-induced diarrhoea. *American Journal of Veterinary Research* **41**, 1039–44.

32 Waterman, A.E. (1984) Practical fluid therapy for small animals. *In Practice* **6**, 143–50.

33 Michell, A.R. (1979) The pathophysiological basis of fluid therapy in small animals. *Veterinary Record* **104**, 542–8.

34 Parry, B.W. (1984) Prognostic evaluation of equine colic cases. *Compendium of Continuing Education for the Practising Veterinarian* **8**, 98–104.

35 Gossett, K.A., Cleghorn, B., Martin, G.S. & Church, G.E. (1987) Correlation between anion gap, blood L-lactate concentration and survival in horses. *Equine Veterinary Journal* **19**, 29–30.

36 Collins, J.A. (1982) Pathophysiology of haemorrhagic shock. In: *Massive Transfusion in Surgery and Trauma*, 5–29. Collins, J.A., Murawski, K. & Shafer, A.W. (eds). A.R. Liss Inc., New York.

37 Cowan, B.N., Burns, H.J.G., Boyle, P. & Ledingham, I. Mc. (1984) The relative prognostic value of lactate and haemodynamic measures in early shock. *Anaesthesia* **39**, 750–5.

38 Parry, B.W., Anderson, G.A. & Gay, C.C. (1983) Prognosis in equine colic: A comparative study of variables used to assess individual cases. *Equine Veterinary Journal* **15**, 211–5.

39 Demling, R.H. & Nerlich, M. (1982) Animal research on hypovolaemic shock. *Progress in Clinical and Biological Research* **108**, 31–50.

40 Cornelius, L.M., Finco, D.R. & Culver, D.H. (1978) Physiologic effects of rapid infusion of Ringer's lactate solution into dogs. *American Journal of Veterinary Research* **39**, 1185–90.

41 Stoddart, J.C. (1984) In: *Trauma and the Anaesthetist*, 13–43. Bailliere Tindall, London.

42 Willats, S.M. (1987) *Lecture Notes on Fluid and Electrolyte Balance*, 155–6. Blackwell Scientific Publications, Oxford.

43 Bowen, J.M. (1980) Are corticosteroids useful in shock therapy? *Journal of the American Veterinary Medical Association* **177**, 453–5.

44 Muir, W.W. (1987) Equine shock: the need for prospective clinical studies. *Equine Veterinary Journal* **19**, 1–7.

Chapter 5
Clinical and laboratory assessment of deficits and disturbances

The diagnosis of a body fluid deficit or a disturbance of fluid balance, like any other diagnosis, is based initially on the case history and the clinical examination of the animal. The importance of the case history cannot be over-emphasized because it can give an excellent broad guide to the probable nature and extent of the deficits or disturbances present and, if the clinical examination suggests that these are correct, treatment can be commenced immediately with reasonable confidence that it will benefit the animal. Later on, the prescribed regime may need to be modified when the results of laboratory examinations become available or the first effects of treatment become obvious, but the impressions gained from an accurate case history are seldom grossly at fault. Thus, cases of derangement of the body fluids can be treated with expectation of success under conditions where sophisticated laboratory results are not available because of the remoteness, delay or the inability to justify expensive laboratory investigations. Laboratory tests may or may not be helpful in diagnosis — their greatest use is in the establishment of base-lines from which the subsequent progress of the individual case can be assessed and in confirming general trends inferred from accumulated experience. Clinical measurements, however, such as those of central venous pressure and of urinary output, can almost invariably be useful guides in the initial assessment of the circulatory state of the animal, as well as for monitoring the progress of treatment. Measurements of arterial pressure are particularly useful in shocked animals but seldom used routinely.

The case history

Important questions to ask

1 Food and fluid intake as assessed by owner.
2 Extent of losses observed by owner: faeces, urine, vomit and blood.

3 Owner's observations of symptoms/behaviour: depression, thirst, faecal consistency and frequency and urinary frequency.

This information can be extremely valuable in setting the stage for the clinical examination to follow. While an observant owner can give all that is required, this may be difficult in some cases where close observation is impeded by circumstances, e.g. farm animals may be observed only infrequently, and cats by their nature keep their personal practices to themselves, so that any estimate of, say faecal losses, may be pure guesswork; moreover injured or sick cats may not return home for several days making any estimate of output or input quite impossible. Dog owners, on the other hand, are often well acquainted (sometimes obsessively) with their pet's urinary and faecal output, and so are a good source of information. However, even here the *volume* lost can be difficult to assess. As with an estimate of blood lost in an accident, a small amount looks impressively large, so a diarrhoeic stool can appear voluminous (particularly on a good carpet). Some dog owners may report that the animal is drinking normally (or excessively) merely because it goes to the bowl without necessarily taking more than a small amount.

Calculations regarding deficits may depend on the species involved. For instance, Tasker [1] has calculated that in the healthy horse there is an additional reserve of about 250 ml/kg of water in the alimentary tract, which is not found in dogs and cats, so that after deprivation of water and food the horse develops a deficit of only about 21 ml/kg/day in spite of a normal daily urinary output until this reserve is also depleted. When intake is curtailed in horses with diarrhoea or intestinal obstruction, however, a large extracellular deficit rapidly develops because of failure to absorb water from the gut.

In drawing up any tentative estimate of probable deficits from the case history it should be remembered that inadequate intake and polyuria usually affect water more than electrolytes. Abnormal losses from the gastrointestinal tract, or internal sequestration of fluid suggest significant deficits of sodium, chloride and potassium ions as well as water, and thus affect circulating volume more readily.

The clinical examination

Although 'dehydration' literally means water depletion, the term is used with wider meaning in clinical practice to describe the signs and symptoms produced by a reduced extracellular fluid volume, i.e. the effects of combined depletion of salt and water. The clinical examination may or may not be helpful since quite severe depletion of the body fluids often produces only minimal clinical signs which are easily missed by even experienced clinicians or confused with signs arising from other causes.

Signs of disturbed water and electrolyte balance

1 Skin turgor — this is most easily tested by taking a pinch of *loose* skin (e.g. flank) and assessing the rate at which the pinch flattens. The eyelid can be used in calves and cattle (Plate 1).
2 Sunken eye — this can be clearly seen in animals where the eye is normally prominent in its setting (e.g. in the calf). It is less clearly visible in a small kitten.
3 Mucous membranes — membranes become sticky and viscid, and as the circulation becomes progressively depressed, cyanosis may become apparent.
4 Respiration rate and depth — metabolic acidosis may be associated with stimulation of respiration in both rate and depth as the animal attempts to excrete CO_2 to correct the blood pH. Conversely, alkalosis leads to respiratory depression although this may not be easy to distinguish clinically.
5 Muscle weakness.
6 Depression.
7 Thirst.

The signs seen in any individual case will depend on the balance of the losses (or excesses) of water and electrolytes, and will probably be complicated by the combination of two or more deficits, since although depletion of water, sodium or potassium produces some characteristic physical signs, most deficits encountered in practice are mixed and these signs tend to become mingled. Nevertheless, it is simpler to consider these phenomena separately, as if they arose from pure depletions of the various constituents of the body fluids.

Water depletion

Thirst is the earliest sign of water depletion. As the water deficit increases, the mucous membranes become dry; this can be detected by touching the tongue and insides of the cheeks with a dry finger, and by examining the conjunctival sacs which appear dry and abnormally red. An animal suffering from advanced water depletion looks weak and ill and behaves in a dull, lethargic manner. There is no marked tachycardia or arterial hypotension until very late in the condition when the blood volume becomes reduced. If electrolytes are measured, hypernatraemia is the cardinal sign. Fever and hot, dry surroundings exacerbate water loss.

Sodium depletion

In sodium depletion (often linked with water loss) clinical signs develop much more rapidly than in water depletion. A sodium depleted animal usually appears very ill and seems to be indifferent to the various procedures involved in the examination. It shows muscular weakness and excessive fatigue when made to stand or walk. The loss of sub-cutaneous fluid produces sunken eyes and a drawn, anxious facial expression. The skin loses its normal turgor and pinched-up skin folds remain 'tented' but the mucous membranes do not become dry. Unless the animal is mouth breathing, the mouth is moist but tacky and the saliva seems viscid. Decreased skin turgor is not as helpful as it is often assumed to be, for changes similar to those seen in extra-cellular fluid depletion occur in wasting diseases unassociated with body fluid depletion. When the decrease in plasma volume becomes severe, the animal passes into oligaemic circulatory failure (shock). In smaller animals impending circulatory failure may sometimes be detected by forced elevation of the head and upper parts of the body. This elevation of the fore-parts of the body seems to make the animal very restless and it struggles, although feebly, until it is allowed to resume a more horizontal posture. In fully developed oligaemic circulatory failure, the skin of the axillae, inside of the thighs and abdomen is clammy, the ears, mouth and feet or hooves are cold to the touch, the mucous membranes pale and sometimes cyanotic. The capillary refill time after blanching by pressure is slow, while the pulse is rapid and of poor volume, 'thready'. The bladder is often empty because the arterial blood pressure has fallen so much that renal function is impaired.

Potassium depletion

Potassium depletion (usually giving a low plasma potassium concentration) produces progressive muscular weakness, intestinal atony and abdominal distension. Cardiac dilatation and failure occur as late features. Plasma concentrations of potassium below about 3.5 mmol/l produce electrocardiographic changes which may be of diagnostic value, with a progressive lowering and broadening of the T-waves, a lengthening of the Q–T interval, depression of the S–T segment (Fig. 5.1) and the appearance of dysrhythmias (ventricular extra-systoles, supraventricular tachycardia, nodal tachycardia, ventricular tachycardia and ventricular fibrillation).

Hypocalcaemia

Hypocalcaemia usually becomes clinically evident when an increased demand is made on calcium resources as in pregnancy and/or lactation or a rise in blood pH suddenly lowers the percentage of ionized calcium. Hypomagnesaemia is so commonly associated with hypo-calcaemia and hypokalaemia that it is often difficult to discern its individual ill-effects. Neither calcium nor magnesium, however, play any major role in body fluid regulation, nor is their correction normally considered part of conventional fluid therapy.

Acid–base disturbance

The principal signs of acid–base disturbances are changes in the character and rate of breathing as respiratory compensatory mechan-isms work to retain or excrete carbon dioxide. In acidosis of metabolic or renal origin, respiratory stimulation occurs and the animal breathes deeply, and often raucously (Kussmaul's breathing), in an attempt to excrete the maximum amount of carbon dioxide to restore the normal blood pH. This type of breathing is perhaps most commonly seen in dogs with severe diabetic ketosis. However, respiratory stimulation is not always detectable even in animals with moderately severe acidosis, especially when the respiratory control mechanisms are depressed by chronic hypoxaemia or toxins. Metabolic alkalosis results in quiet, shallow breathing, usually indistinguishable from normal breathing at rest. An apparent decrease in the rate and depth of breathing during treatment may be the result of an induced alkalosis but is more likely to be attributable to other causes such as the restoration of the circulating fluid volume.

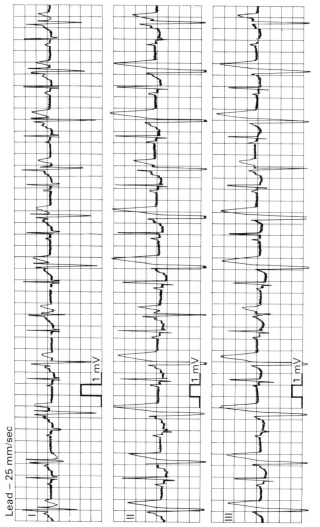

Fig. 5.1 ECG from a dog with plasma K^+ 2.2 mmol/l (hypokalaemia). The most prominent feature is the alternation of ventricular extrasystoles with normally triggered QRS complexes (bigeminy).

Excess water/electrolytes

Excesses of water and electrolytes in the body are usually iatrogenic. Water excess, i.e. hyponatraemia, is not well tolerated because it causes cells to swell and the extent to which the brain can swell without symptomatic rise in intracranial pressure is small because the brain is enclosed in the rigid cranium. The animal becomes restless, then dull and finally comatose. Muscle twitching or fibrillation may also be seen. The signs of saline excess include an increase in body weight due to water retention, increased jugular venous pressure and, later, oedema with pulmonary crepitations and radiological evidence of septal oedema and pleural effusions. The effect of excess salt ingestion is to cause hypernatraemia but only if the animal is unable to drink. Acute changes in plasma sodium concentration of the order of 15 mmol/l are likely to cause behavioural symptoms but greater changes may have less effect if they are gradual [2]. Hyperkalaemia can occur despite a net potassium loss where potassium moves extracellularly and enters the blood with a metabolic acidosis. It is symptomless until extreme (over about 8 mmol/l) when it causes weakness and extreme mental agitation. Disorders of the heart rate and rhythm develop before other signs become obvious and ventricular fibrillation or standstill is the final and fatal cardiac manifestation of hyperkalaemia. Although electrolyte disturbances cause clinical signs, they are seldom distinctive of a specific abnormality.

Mixed deficits

Clearly, the physical effects of a mixed depletion will depend on the ratio of water to electrolyte lost and the renal and thirst responses; thus a variety of clinical states can occur. As a general guide, however, dry mucous membranes, oliguria and thirst point to a predominantly water depletion, while tachycardia, moist or tacky mucous membranes, poor skin turgor and 'postural discomfort' are the principal features of predominantly electrolyte depletions. So effective is the healthy kidney in excreting and conserving both water and electrolytes that only the most extreme variations are harmful. However, the time taken to reach the critical state is much less in small or immature animal patients than larger ones because the initial reserves are much smaller, whereas the losses may remain disproportionately large. A rough but useful estimate of the extent of a deficit may be possible from certain clinical signs (Table 5.1).

Table 5.1 Degree of dehydration and associated symptoms

Fluid deficit (% of BWt)	Symptom
0−5%	No clear symptom (thirst) (depression)
5−7%	Skin elasticity lowered (tenting), sunken eye, cold nose
7−10%	Collapse, cold extremities, pulse weak
10−12%	Progressive shock

This 'rule of thumb' guide seems not to be based on any scientific investigations but has been accepted as reasonably reliable by clinicians for many years. It at least reminds us that deficits requiring correction are unlikely to be less than 40 ml/kg or more than 150 ml/kg. Occasionally even greater deficits are encountered, especially in calves [3].

Laboratory examinations

Urinalysis

Analysis of blood and urine samples collected at the time of the initial examination can provide information which may assist both in reinforcing the first assessment of the state of the animal's hydration and in judgement of progress during treatment. Since the kidney may sometimes be the cause of the body fluid disturbance or, more usually, may be responding to correct the upset with varying success, interpretation of results obtained from urine can be extremely difficult.

In predominant water depletion in otherwise healthy animals the urine is highly concentrated while the plasma osmolality, plasma sodium and albumin concentrations, the haemoglobin concentration and haematocrit (PCV) are raised. In water excess the urine will be very dilute, the plasma osmolality reduced, and the haemoglobin concentration and PCV low. The principal findings in saline (extra-cellular fluid) depletion are very concentrated but almost sodium-free urine. Renal conservation of sodium is normally so effective that it is almost impossible to induce symptomatic sodium deficiency by any reduction in the sodium intake unaccompanied by abnormal loss as occurs in vomiting. Animals with chronic renal disease, however, neither conserve nor eliminate sodium normally and are unable to reduce their urinary excretion of sodium rapidly in response to a lowered intake.

The concentrating ability of the kidneys is usually assessed from the specific gravity of the urine which is generally a fair indicator of the concentration of solutes present and thus of urine osmolality. The correlation between specific gravity and osmolality may, however, be very poor in oliguric states or if the urine contains abnormal constituents. Thus, it is most important to test the urine for the presence of abnormal constituents such as protein and glucose which will make specific gravity measurement an unreliable guide to kidney function. Proteinuria may be post-renal in origin and microscopic examination of urinary deposit is useful in revealing the source of the protein.

Measurement of urinary pH may provide information about the acid—base status of the animal, although when the kidneys are normal, small changes may be obscured by the operation of renal buffering mechanisms. Generally, however, in the absence of renal disease, changes in urinary pH may be taken to reflect the relative quantities of hydrogen ions being excreted unless the need to retain potassium and sodium has overridden the maintenance of normal acid—base balance. Thus, in the metabolic alkalosis which follows vomiting, hydrogen ions are excreted in exchange for sodium ions giving rise to the paradox of an acid urine in the presence of a metabolic alkalosis (Chapter 2). Urine pH may also be affected by infections of the urinary tract or by the excretion of certain drugs in the urine. In any case, measurements of urinary pH only serve as indications that an acid—base disturbance is likely to be present; they do not indicate the degree of the disturbance. As in most clinical situations, serial measurements are more informative than initial or isolated ones and are useful in monitoring the response to measures designed to correct the acid—base status of the animal, e.g. over-correction of metabolic acidosis, leading to alkaline urine.

Even where facilities exist for the analysis of electrolytes in the urine, it is wise not to attribute too much importance to the results obtained. Measurement of 24-hour urinary excretion of electrolytes is generally of no value since the intake is seldom known and the loss by other normal and abnormal routes is unmeasured. In the ideal situation, when the intake is known and there are no abnormal losses other than the small daily loss in faeces and sweat, the imbalance between intake and output may still be so small as to be within the limits of experimental error in collection and estimation. This is not to say, however, that this difference in intake and output may not, as a cumulative imbalance, cause disease.

Blood samples [4]

Examination of the blood must be regarded as being of primary importance in the management of disturbances of fluid and electrolyte balance and serial estimations yield the greatest value because they enable the response to treatment to be monitored. A blood sample should be taken before treatment is started, or very shortly afterwards. When fluids are to be administered by the intravenous route it is often convenient to sample blood through the intravenous catheter through which the fluids will be given, so sparing the animal an additional venepuncture. In a severely hypotensive animal, collection of venous blood in this manner may be the only practical procedure. Determination of *packed cell volume* (PCV) and *total plasma protein concentration* are the usual measurements made.

In the early stages of fluid depletion, changes in PCV may be small due to the operation of homeostatic mechanisms which tend to maintain the intravascular volume at the expense of the other body fluid compartments. The PCV will become increased when loss of isotonic fluid reduces the plasma volume but in a predominantly water depletion, shrinkage of the red cells may mask an increase in PCV. In cases of predominantly sodium depletion, the red cells will swell so that the PCV will appear to be high giving a false impression of water loss. Obviously, any deductions from the PCV regarding fluid problems are of value only if the PCV before the upset is known. Reliability of PCV values will also be affected by ease of sampling and, especially in dogs and sheep, by splenic contraction induced by stress.

Estimation of *haemoglobin concentration* is generally less rapid than that of PCV so that PCV measurement is usually preferred but combination of these two determinations can provide very useful additional information. In water deprivation, where the cells shrink and the PCV rises due to reduction in plasma water so that a near normal PCV may be found, a high haemoglobin concentration relative to the PCV will reveal the true state of water depletion. Conversely, in the case of predominantly sodium depletion the haemoglobin concentration will be low relative to the observed PCV [5].

Calculation of the *mean corpuscular haemoglobin, mean corpuscular haemoglobin concentration* and *mean corpuscular volume* from the red cell count and PCV will always reveal the presence of red cell shrinkage or swelling, whether this is due to water or sodium depletion or to some type of anaemia. However, red cell counts are tedious to perform unless an expensive cell counter is available. It is, therefore, more usual to check on interpretation of PCV estimations by determination of the *total plasma protein* content because the value of this will be unaffected by shifts of water from the extracellular to intracellular fluids in the same way that PCV would be affected. Contraction of plasma water volume is always associated with a rise in total plasma proteins to above the normal level unless hypoproteinaemia was present before the disturbance of fluid balance developed or the pathological fluid loss is rich in protein, e.g. protein-losing enteropathy.

Plasma sodium and potassium (Figures 5.2 and 5.3)

Plasma electrolyte estimations are but poor guides to the extent of total body losses. If any electrolyte deficit is accompanied by simultaneous water loss resulting in contraction of the extracellular volume, the plasma concentration of the electrolyte will depend not only on that electrolyte, but also on the extent of the contraction in the plasma volume. Moreover, plasma sodium concentration primarily reflects water balance and plasma potassium, which is certainly important, may change independent of cell potassium (Chapter 2). Clinical assessment of evidence for fluid depletion or excess is fundamental to the interpretation of plasma sodium concentration (and hence plasma osmolality). For example, if a hyponatraemic animal shows signs of volume depletion and the urine is virtually sodium-free, indicating a normal response to sodium deficiency, the animal is either suffering from salt and water loss by an extra-renal route such as the gastrointestinal tract or from a severe restriction of intake. A higher urinary sodium in these circumstances indicates failure of normal renal conservation of this electrolyte either due to renal or adrenal disease. Probably the most important information to be derived from plasma electrolyte determinations alone comes from estimation of potassium levels, for hypokalaemia indicates that the very large intracellular stores of this electrolyte have been severely

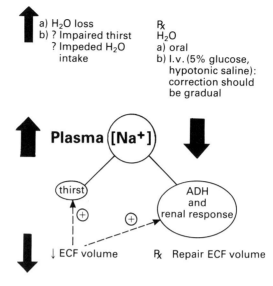

Fig. 5.2 Plasma sodium: main disturbances and their correction.

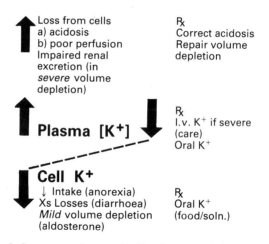

Fig. 5.3 Cell and plasma potassium: main disturbances and their correction.

depleted and urgent steps need to be taken to restore the concentration to within the normal range. Moreover, the effects of hypokalaemia or hyperkalaemia are potentially serious, regardless of their cause. Fortunately, some of the newer kit-analysers are starting to include potassium in their range. Quantitative assessment of cell K^+, using RBC, is only really applicable in horses and is discussed in Chapter 6.

Acid—base evaluation

Acid—base balance has a long history of clinical confusion and in veterinary practice lack of easily available facilities for its investigation have contributed to its generally being excluded from consideration of fluid and electrolyte disturbances. Nevertheless, metabolic acidosis remains potentially lethal. Recent years have seen a change as more centres have become equipped with the expensive, sophisticated apparatus needed for acid—base studies, i.e. for the direct measurement of pH and Pco_2 by ion-selective electrodes. In anaerobically sampled and stored arterial blood a pH outside the range of about $7.15-7.5$ indicates potential danger to life and justifies therapeutic intervention, especially if the derangement is acute. Since pH is proportional to the log. of the HCO_3/Pco_2 ratio, pH and Pco_2 measurements allow bicarbonate to be calculated and, usually, expressed as departure from normal (base deficit, base excess) in mmol/l. Though based on human or canine data [6, 7], such approximations are more than adequate for clinical decisions.

Determination of the pH of venous blood is meaningless as far as respiratory acid—base disturbances are concerned since its CO_2 particularly reflects metabolic activity in the tissues drained by the vein from which the blood is drawn. It must always be remembered that an arterial blood pH within the normal range for the species of animal by no means precludes alkalosis or acidosis or even the presence of both, i.e. of compensated or mixed disturbances (Chapter 2). Because the clinical signs of acid—base disturbances are so vague [3], laboratory investigations carried out on anaerobically drawn blood samples are essential for correct diagnosis.

Very recently it has been shown that, rather than being expensive and almost unobtainable, acid—base estimations could become a rapid, inexpensive routine measurement in the veterinary practice laboratory. The 'gold-standard' of acid—base evaluation has always been the Van Slyke technique even though it was too cumbersome for routine clinical use. A very similar approach has been available for some time in the form of a simple kit, intended for use with serum, and measuring TCO_2 (Fig. 5.4). Hitherto it has had little impact in veterinary medicine. An evaluation in calf diarrhoea now shows that this instrument is capable, when correctly used, of high precision, by clinical standards, thus allowing acid—base status to be determined with reasonable confidence from samples of venous whole blood [8].

For classification of metabolic acid–base disturbances into alkalosis, normality, mild, moderate or severe acidosis, the inaccuracies introduced by the use of venous blood are trivial and such samples have the decisive advantage that, being routine, they will actually be taken. Anaerobic sampling is simple (exclusion or rapid expulsion of bubbles) and storage precautions need no more than ice and polystyrene, if analysis is postponed. Since the kit is small, immediate analysis 'in car' within minutes is feasible but the routine laboratory is likely to provide a better setting for precision.

The test converts the blood bicarbonate to CO_2 with acid which also liberates the CO_2 carried in the blood. Since the latter normally yields only 5% of the total yield of gas on acidification (Chapter 2), TCO_2 is primarily a measure of blood bicarbonate, i.e. metabolic acidosis or alkalosis. The influence of changes in P_{CO_2} is trivial, especially when it is borne in mind that formulae for replacement of the deficit vary greatly as to whether the volume of body fluid needing additional bicarbonate corresponds to the ECF or something more, to allow for H^+ held by intracellular buffers [9]. Thus the ECF space is about 20% of body weight but it is usually assumed that the space in which a base deficit needs to be corrected corresponds to 30–50% of body weight, generally 30%.

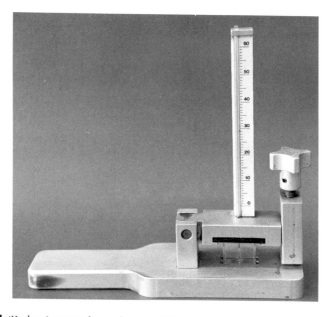

Fig. 5.4 'Harleco' system for acid–base (TCO_2) measurements.

The kit is, of course, inferior to a blood gas analysis, especially as respiratory compensation for the disturbance cannot be judged, nor the existence of concurrent respiratory disturbances which may influence treatment, e.g. a respiratory alkalosis complicating metabolic acidosis. For the majority, however, who until now have had nothing to guide their decision except history and judgement, it is a luxury to worry about such shortcomings. Moreover, TCO_2 samples are more robust than blood gas analysis when the influence of sample storage artefacts is considered [10].

Anion gap

A subsidiary component of acid–base evaluation which is very useful in man and has started to be appreciated in veterinary medicine, especially equine medicine, is 'anion gap' [11, 12] (Chapter 2).

If all the conveniently measurable anions and cations in plasma are added up, the total concentration of cations exceeds that of anions by some 20–30 mmol/l. Since the main cations are Na and K this calculation is best expressed as:

$$[Na + K] - [Cl + HCO_3] = a$$

where a = anion gap.

The gap reflects organic anions such as lactate and others — hence interpretation may be difficult if solutions with bicarbonate precursors have been given. Simply, however, in a metabolic acidosis caused by bicarbonate loss the kidney, being short of bicarbonate, tends to accompany sodium by chloride instead, i.e. anion gap is unchanged since bicarbonate and chloride undergo reciprocal change. Where the problem is accumulation of acid, e.g. during lactic acidosis associated with ischaemia or following excess grain consumption and fermentation, the anion gap increases as the bicarbonate falls; chloride tends to stay unaltered. In shock associated with equine colic, anion gap may have great prognostic value [13].

Osmolality [14, 15]

Essentially, this gives the same information as measurements of plasma sodium concentration, i.e. it helps to distinguish between hypertonic and hypotonic dehydration or to indicate excess water

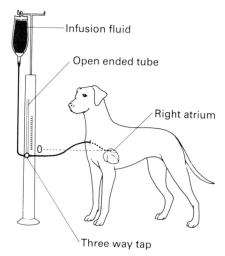

Fig. 5.5 Simplified diagram of equipment for measuring CVP in a dog, using a saline manometer.

retention. It can be calculated by summing the mOsm of the major solutes, i.e. electrolytes + glucose and urea, and a good approximation comes from:

Osmolality (mOsm/l) = 2 [Na + K] + glucose + urea (all in mmol/l).

More satisfactorily, it is measured directly using an osmometer, but cost makes this a procedure for the professional laboratory. The machines read directly and mostly work on the principle of freezing point depression being related to osmolar concentration.

Measurement of the central venous pressure (Fig. 5.5)

The height of the jugular venous pressure in the standing animal or in the sternally recumbent animal is a useful indicator of the plasma volume and of the presence or absence of right heart failure. Precise measurement of central venous pressure (CVP) by a central venous catheter is particularly useful in guiding the rate and volume of fluid replacement in acute illness provided care is taken to avoid obvious pitfalls such as blocked or malpositioned catheters and to interpret the findings in the context of the whole clinical picture.

Central venous pressure gives an indication of both right ventricular function and of plasma volume. Impairment of right ventricular function and expansion of the plasma volume cause the measured pressure to rise while deficiency of extracellular fluid will result in a lowered pressure. This does not, however, mean that replacement of plasma volume can be planned by reference to the CVP alone because left ventricular failure (which is insensitively monitored by the CVP) may precede the full correction of plasma volume depletion. CVP may also rise prematurely during rehydration, due to sustained venocon- striction, e.g. in a shocked animal which is still volume depleted. A significant sustained rise of CVP implies a risk of pulmonary oedema, partly because it suggests cardiac overload but also because it impedes pulmonary lymphatic drainage [16]. It is also important to realize that salt and water replacement in a dehydrated animal cannot easily be judged from the CVP if the plasma albumin concentration is low — the plasma volume may be low because oncotic pressure is reduced and plasma volume cannot be restored to normal by the administration of electrolyte solutions without, at the same time, risking peripheral and pulmonary oedema. In addition, the CVP is an insensitive marker of absolute water excess or deficiency because plasma volume is affected proportionately with all the body fluids, i.e. sustains the minority of the total deficit (Chapter 2).

Trends in the CVP shown by serial determinations are more sig- nificant than single values and although low values for CVP may be obtained in some normally hydrated animals, a low reading usually indicates a need for volume replacement. A useful diagnostic technique is to infuse about 1 ml/kg of blood, plasma or plasma substitute over a period of 2 minutes. This should cause an initial rise in CVP which will soon return to its original level after the infusion is slowed or stopped if there is a reduction in circulating blood volume. If the induced rise in CVP persists, either there is no plasma deficit or the right heart is failing and caution must be exercised in the rate of any further infusion which is judged to be necessary on other grounds. It is important to note that there are major differences in the CVP levels recorded in different species and that correct 'zeroing' is essential for reliable CVP measurements.

Accurate measurement of CVP requires jugular catheterization. Ideally, the tip of the catheter should be advanced to lie adjacent to but not in the right atrium. For clinical use, however, particularly in small animals, results obtained using short catheters may be adequate. The venous pressure can then be monitored using a saline man- ometer (Fig. 5.5) or with an aneroid system such as the 'Pressurveil' (Plate 2).

When taking readings, the zero of the manometer must be level with the right atrium. Unfortunately, it is not possible to judge this position easily and a variety of external markers have been suggested for the zero position; these include the tip of the sternum and the point of the shoulder. It is probable that none of these maintains a constant relationship to the position of the heart when the animal is placed in different positions. The associated error may only be 1−2 cm (aqueous solution) in small animals but is considerably greater in horses and cattle. This error probably explains many of the aberrant results which occur with CVP measurements, and the differences between stated normal values. The important priorities are to use a consistent technique and to pay attention to changes as well as absolute levels. We would expect CVPs in normal dogs and cats to be around 2−4 cm (aqueous) and in a dehydrated animal values below zero are likely [17]. A rise of 6 cm should cause reduction of administration rate. The sources of variation in the horse make it much harder to give unqualified statements as to exact values [18].

References

1 Tasker, J.B. (1967) Fluid and electrolyte studies in the horse. *Cornell Veterinarian* **57**, 649−77.

2 Michell, A.R. (1979) Biochemistry and behaviour: systemic aspects of neurological disturbances. *Journal of Small Animal Practice* **20**, 645−9.

3 Groutides, C.P. (1988) Studies of fluid, electrolyte and acid−base balance in diarrhoiec calves with special reference to fluid therapy. PhD Thesis, University of London.

4 Kerr, M.G. (1988) *Veterinary Laboratory Medicine: Haematology and Clinical Chemistry.* Blackwell Scientific Publications, Oxford.

5 Michell, A.R. (1968) Fluid therapy for calves. *Veterinary Record* **82**, 517.

6 Puschett, J.B. & Piraino, B. (1985) Disorders of acid−base balance. In: *Disorders of Fluid and Electrolyte Balance*, 1−38. Puschett, J.B. (ed). Churchill Livingstone, New York.

7 Clark, C.H. (1981) Fluid therapy. In: *Veterinary Critical Care*, 415−34. Sattler, F.D., Knowles, R.P. & Whittick, W.G. (eds). Lea & Febiger, Philadelphia.

8 Groutides, C. & Michell, A.R. (1988) A method for assessment of acid−base disturbances. *Clinical Insight* **3**, 209−10.

9 Rose, B.D. (1977) *Clinical Physiology of Acid−Base and Electrolyte Disorders*, 323−54. McGraw Hill, New York.

10 Rispens, P. (1981) Determination of total carbon dioxide. In: *Blood pH, Carbon Dioxide, Oxygen and Calcium Ions*, 52−5. Siggard-Andersen, O. (ed). Private Press, Copenhagen.

11 Polzin, D.J. & Osborne, C.A. (1986) Anion gap — diagnostic and therapeutic applications. In: *Current Veterinary Therapy IX*, 52−9. Kirk, R.W. (ed). W.B. Saunders, Philadelphia.

12 Carroll, H.J. & Oh, M.S. (1978) *Water, Electrolyte and Acid−Base Metabolism: Diagnosis and Management*, 246−52. J.B. Lippincott, Philadelphia.

13 Gossett, K.A., Cleghorn, B., Martin, G.S. & Church, G.E. (1987) Correlation between anion gap, blood L-lactate concentration and survival in horses. *Equine Veterinary Journal* **19**, 29−30.

14 Willatts, S.M. (1987) *Lecture Notes on Fluid and Electrolyte Balance*, 11−15. Blackwell Scientific Publications, Oxford.

15 Brownlow, M.A. & Hutchins, D.R. (1982) The concept of osmolality: its use in the evaluation of 'dehydration' in the horse. *Equine Veterinary Journal* **14**, 106−10. (See also Muylle E. & Van den Hende, C.; Comments in *Equine Veterinary Journal* **15**, 80−1.)

16 Allen, S.J., Draker, R.E., Williams, J.P., Laine, G.A. & Gabel, J.C. (1987) Recent advances in pulmonary oedema. *Critical Care Medicine* **15**, 923−9.

17 Hall, L.W. (1967) *Fluid Balance in Canine Surgery*, 44. Bailliere, London.

18 Schatzmann, U. & Battier, R. (1987) Some experiences with central venous pressure (CVP) measurements in the horse. *Journal of the Association of Veterinary Anaesthetists* **14**, 109.

Chapter 6
Quantitative aspects of fluid therapy

The alternative title of this chapter might be: 'How much (and how fast)?' but the answer to this question is almost impossible to formulate simply, since requirements depend so much on the size of the animal and the nature of the illness. In veterinary practice we deal most of the time with volume depletion states and therefore in deciding volume requirements we need to make some estimate of the deficit which the animal has accumulated.

Methods of estimating the size of volume deficit

The two main ways of estimating the size of volume deficit are:
1 The 'factorial' approach, based on net deficits resulting from:
a Abnormal losses.
b Failure of intake to match normal losses.
2 The 'clinical' approach, based essentially on the animal's history and appearance.

Factorial

Dr L.W. Hall [1] developed a way of using a knowledge of normal fluid intake combined with obtaining an accurate history of the duration and nature of the illness in each patient. This method is described by Waterman [2] and has proved entirely satisfactory in the authors' experience.

The following is an example of calculating fluid requirements.

History

A 20 kg female dog inappetant for 3 days and vomiting profusely once daily since the onset of the illness. Urinating decreased in frequency for last 2 days. This dog has a high intestinal FB.

Calculation

1 25 ml/kg/day three days'
  inevitable water loss at $\qquad$ (3 × 20 × 25) = 1500 ml
2 25 ml/kg/day one day's
  urinary water loss at $\qquad$ (1 × 20 × 25) = 500 ml
3 4 ml/kg vomit losses in
  vomiting at $\qquad$ (4 × 20 × 1 × 3) = 240 ml

$\qquad$ Total deficit $\qquad$ = 2240 ml
$\qquad$ ECF deficit (33%) $\qquad$ = 750 ml
$\qquad$ Plasma deficit (25% of ECF) = 190 ml

This dog therefore needs approximately 200 ml rapidly to support its circulation and a further 2 l given slowly to replenish the rest of the deficit during and after surgery.

Clinical

The alternative approach, often adopted in North America, depends solely on physical examination of the animal. Cornelius [3] described this approach which involves examination of the texture and elasticity of the skin and the appearance of the mucous membranes. He suggests that signs to be looked for include loss of elasticity and pliability of the skin, depression of the eye into the orbit and dryness of the oral mucosa. He states that clinical evidence of dehydration is not present if water losses are less than 5% of body weight, and at the other extreme losses greater than 15% are usually incompatible with life. Consequently, estimates of dehydration are always between 5 and 15%. Table 6.2 indicates the relative changes Cornelius [3] records with increasing degrees of dehydration.

However, there are many pitfalls with this approach (Chapter 5). The major one is that animals suffering a primary water loss tend not to show these 'classical signs' of dehydration and so one can be entirely misled. Secondly, even if the animal is suffering from a mixed electrolyte and water depletion, the following caveats apply:
1 Cachetic animals' skin loses elasticity because of fat and protein even when they are not dehydrated.
2 Fat animals' skin tends to retain elasticity even though the animal may be dehydrated.

This approach, therefore, can only ever give a very rough estimate of fluid requirements since it is impossible to detect, clinically, a 1%

Table 6.1 Changes with increasing degrees of dehydration

% Dehydration	Signs
<5%	Undetectable clinically
5%	Skin begins to feel doughy
7%	Skin loses elasticity, eye sunk into orbit. Capillary refill time prolonged
10−12%	Changes more pronounced. May also show signs of hypovolaemic shock
12−15%	Moribund

difference in dehydration, i.e. the difference between 5 and 6% or 8 and 9% dehydration. It may also underestimate some of the severer deficits, particularly in calves (Chapter 5).

The technique does have its advocates, however, and at least for large animal work, it provides a reminder of the magnitude of deficits encountered, for example: a 500 kg cow which is 10% dehydrated will require

$$500 \times \frac{10}{100} = 50 \text{ l}$$

It should be noted that '% dehydration' describes the percentage loss of body weight attributed to dehydration, not the percentage of body water lost. As in all measurements of body fluid compartments during dehydration, the baseline is the measured or assumed *normal* body weight, *prior* to dehydration.

Other methods of estimating the size of the deficits are based on:
1 Body weight.
2 Laboratory aids.
3 Acid−base requirements.
4 Osmolality of blood.

Body weight

A knowledge of the animal's body weight before the onset of the illness can be useful since acute loss of weight is usually almost entirely due to dehydration. Monitoring body weight during an illness can also give valuable information on fluid requirements but one should also remember that tissue catabolism may be going on as well and may be responsible for some of the weight loss. This may be considerable in calves [4].

Laboratory aids

Packed cell volume and total proteins both rise as a result of dehydration but it is important to perform both tests to minimize the risk of misinterpretation of data because of pre-existing abnormalities. For instance, a pre-existing anaemia or hypoproteinaemia will affect the readings considerably and splenic contraction in response to sympatho-adrenal stimulation will increase the PCV, even in the absence of dehydration.

A very rough estimate of volume requirements may be made from the PCV alone. There are several formulae published which vary according to whether the deficit is assumed to be extracellular or shared throughout the whole body. A common formula, assuming the deficit is extracellular, is to allow 10 ml/kg body weight for each 1% rise in PCV above 'normal'.

If A = normal body weight (kg), *B* = dehydrated PCV (%), and *C* = normal PCV (%):

$$\text{Deficit in plasma volume} = 100\,A\left(1 - \frac{C}{B}\right) \text{ (Chapter 5, [5])}$$

Thus if PCV rises by 1, and *A* = 1 kg:

$$\text{Deficit in plasma volume} = 100\left(1 - \frac{46}{45}\right)$$

$$= 2.222\,\text{ml/kg}$$

Therefore, ECF deficit = 8.888 ml/kg, i.e. approximately 10 ml/kg for a PCV increase of 1.

A more accurate estimate can be made by utilizing the total protein (TP) figures also, as a cross-check.

If M and *N* = measured and normal TP, and *R* and *V* = reduced and normal plasma volume, *then MR* = *VN and* $\dfrac{R}{V} = \dfrac{N}{M}$

Thus % fall in plasma volume (*D*) = $100 - \left(\dfrac{R}{V} \times 100\right)$

$$= 100 - \left(\frac{N}{M} \times 100 \right)$$

This % deficit (D) is assumed to apply to the entire ECF (20% body weight) for isotonic losses, entire body water (60% body weight) for predominant water loss.

$$\textit{Thus} \text{ total deficit} = \text{BWt} \times \frac{20}{100} \times \frac{D}{100}$$

$$\textit{or} \qquad\qquad = \text{BWt} \times \frac{60}{100} \times \frac{D}{100}$$

Obviously, dehydration is not the only factor affecting total protein, e.g. a protein-losing enteropathy will tend to reduce it.

Plasma electrolyte concentrations are of limited value as estimates of the whole body status of each ion. Low levels of any electrolyte usually indicate a large deficit which requires urgent correction, but normal plasma levels do not rule out a deficit. High Na^+ and Cl^- usually indicate a primary water deficit.

Acid–base requirements

The bicarbonate deficit in plasma may be measured either by the use of a blood gas machine or by measuring TCO_2 (Chapter 5).

Bicarbonate requirements may be determined by using the following formula:

$$('Normal' - measured) \times \frac{\text{BWt (kg)}}{3}$$

The term ('normal' – measured) is the approximate 'base deficit' in mmol/l. (It is more common to think of base excess (measured – normal) but this is inconvenient since the common acid–base disturbance, metabolic acidosis, is then expressed as a negative base excess.)

In the absence of such measurements, it is useful to reflect that administration of sufficient bicarbonate to raise plasma bicarbonate by 10 mmol/l will convert a severe acidosis to a mild one but will not dangerously over-correct a mild acidosis. Estimates of the volume of the body fluid requiring additional bicarbonate vary and some believe that only the ECF deficit should be corrected, which represents only

20% of body weight (200 ml/kg); most, however, take account of the need to allow for the H^+ temporarily buffered within the cells too, hence the 33% of body weight in the above formula. As with all volume replacement, the safe approach is initially to replace only *half* the estimated deficit and to monitor progress before giving the rest — i.e. 3.3 mmol/kg is the body 'bicarbonate deficit' implied by a measured base deficit of 10 mmol/l and the *initial* therapy, to replace half, would be 1.6 mmol/kg.

In the absence of facilities for blood gas analysis, inferences may be drawn from other changes. Urine pH in dogs and cats is often affected by acid–base status so that very low or high levels may be of clinical significance. However, this relationship is not invariable and results must be interpreted with extreme care.

The presence of an increased anion gap (Chapter 5) may serve as a useful indicator of the presence of a lactic acidosis caused by hypovolaemic shock. Similarly, high K^+ levels are often found in conjunction with a metabolic acidosis and these laboratory findings can give one a high index of suspicion that metabolic disturbances are present.

Osmolality

In recent years interest has grown in measuring the osmolality of blood, in order to give more information as to whether the animal is suffering from hypo or hypertonic dehydration (Chapters 2 and 5).

Developing a plan

A standard approach to estimating fluid volume needs is important if one is to be successful in meeting the animal's needs. There are three distinct phases to treatment:
1 Correction of the existing deficit.
2 Meeting normal daily requirements.
3 Replacing ongoing abnormal losses.

Correction of the existing deficit

This has two phases:
1 Restoration of the circulating blood volume.
2 Replenishing the rest of the loss.

Restoration of the circulating blood volume to normal is always the first consideration in all cases of fluid depletion. The volume of fluid required can be calculated from the estimated plasma deficit (which is 8% of the total deficit if one assumes that any loss has been equally shared throughout the body). This assumes predominant water loss; in isotonic loss, ECF sustains the entire deficit and plasma 25% of it (see p. 105 for worked example). The change in PCV and TP levels *may* be used as a guide (see above).

Ideally, the fluid used to repair the circulating blood volume deficit in shock should be plasma or a plasma substitute. The rate of infusion can be very fast particularly with crystalloids; in animals with no pre-existing renal or cardiovascular disease, a rate of 90 ml/kg/hour can safely be tolerated for the first 30 minutes to 1 hour [5]. Obviously, this flow rate will replace the whole circulating blood volume within 1 hour and therefore is not recommended to be continued for longer than is needed to improve the animal's cardiovascular status. Generally, if rough estimates cannot be calculated, approximately 5−10 ml/kg of a colloid solution may be given quickly over 20−30 minutes in order to improve the animal's condition and then the infusion may be changed to a crystalloid solution infused at a slower rate.

Replenishing the rest of the deficit. This can be made up more *slowly* than the plasma deficit. Once the circulation improves, the fluid infused should be changed to a crystalloid solution and the infusion rate slowed to allow for replacing the total deficit over 24−48 hours with 50% being given in the first 6 hours or so at the rate of 5−10 ml/kg/hour, and progress being monitored [5]. Thus, the dog in the worked example would receive 180−200 ml of colloid rapidly (over 30 minutes this would work out at 20 ml/kg/hour) and of the remaining 2l, 1 litre would be given over 6 hours — i.e. at around 8 ml/kg/hour — and the second l would be given over the next 18 hours together with the daily maintenance requirements for that day.

Meeting normal daily requirements

Normal daily needs vary between 40 and 50 ml/kg but in most species, they tend to increase in illness and up to twice this may be required, depending on urine output. These volumes must be supplied daily until the animal is able and willing to drink voluntarily again.

Maintenance solutions are hypotonic, e.g. N/5 saline with 4.3% dextrose (Chapter 3).

Replacing ongoing abnormal losses

The volume of continuing abnormal losses can be estimated by the clinician and this amount must be added to the normal daily requirement to give the total daily volume. It may be possible to measure losses exactly (pleural, peritoneal effusions) but often in vomiting and diarrhoea only a 'guesstimate' can be made. Vomiting losses for instance may be conservatively estimated at 1 ml/kg/vomit while diarrhoea accounts for losses of up to 200 ml/kg/day.

Rate of infusion

There is no hard and fast rule governing the rate of infusion. In animals suffering from hypovolaemic shock, the fluid replacement needs to be as fast as possible and several veins may be cannulated simultaneously whereas in small dogs with a moderate deficit the infusion rate must be slower. In hypovolaemic shock an infusion rate of 3 ml/kg/minute for the first 20 minutes or so can be used until the animal's condition improves. In less severely affected animals an infusion rate of 10–15 ml/kg/hour will allow rapid rehydration. For administering normal maintenance requirements, a rate of 5 ml/kg/hour is ideal but often not practicable since it would necessitate giving fluids over 10 hours and usually a faster infusion rate is employed (10 ml/kg/hour).

The flow rate per hour can be converted to drops per minute by using the following formula:

$$\text{Drops/minute} = \frac{\text{drops/ml}}{60} \times \text{ml/kg BWt} \times \text{BWt in kg}$$

Thus a flow rate of 10 ml/kg/hour for a 12 kg dog using a giving set which delivers 15 drops/ml will be:

$$\frac{15}{60} \times 10 \times 12 = 30 \text{ drops/minute}$$

When to stop

In dogs suffering from mild to moderate dehydration, with no preexisting renal or cardiovascular disease, an infusion rate of up to

360 ml/kg of crystalloids for one hour produced no more than mild signs of pulmonary oedema, nasal discharge and elevation of CVP and pulmonary wedge pressure [6]. While an infusion of 90 ml/kg over 1 hour had no deleterious effect [7], greater caution is required in cats, and rates above 40–50 ml/kg/hour are probably a risk [8, 9]. In large animals, practicality usually restricts the use of very high infusion rates.

Nonetheless, there are tell-tale signs that the infusion rate or the volume given is perhaps excessive and when they are detected, the infusion should be slowed. These include the development of moist rales on auscultation and the presence of a moist cough or a serous nasal discharge. Venous congestion especially of the jugular vein and a sustained rise in CVP (Chapter 5) should also be taken as signs that the infusion should be slowed or stopped. These warn of impending pulmonary oedema whereas clinical signs appear only when it is advanced.

Urine output is a useful indicator of renal perfusion and should increase once circulation improves. If, after initial resuscitation, urine output is not restored, then the infusion must be slowed if dangerous pulmonary oedema is to be avoided.

Potassium

In animals suffering from profuse vomiting, protracted diarrhoea or prolonged anorexia, potassium reserves are depleted, even if initially plasma levels are normal. If plasma levels fall, clinical signs of hypokalaemia will become evident and specific therapy will be essential. Mild hypokalaemia may be treated (in suitable cases) by oral supplementation with potassium gluconate. Levels below 3.00 mmol/l in the vomiting/anorexic animal usually require parenteral therapy. If giving K^+-containing fluids intravenously it is the *rate* of administration which is critical; it is unwise to exceed an infusion rate of 0.5 mmol/kg/hour. Since fluids are given at about 10–15 ml/kg/hour this means that the potassium concentration should not exceed 30 mmol/l in order to avoid any potentially dangerous surge in plasma potassium levels.

The total amount of potassium required to restore body deficits can only be estimated if one attempts to measure intracellular K^+ as described by Muylle *et al.* [10]. Most of our species are unusual in having RBC with low K^+. Thus, it is only of potential clinical use in the horse and as a more general guide it is recommended that a total dose of 5 mmol K^+/kg/24 hours is not exceeded.

Acid—base imbalances

If a blood gas machine or TCO_2 kit is available, calculation of the amount of bicarbonate required is fairly straightforward using the formula already given (p. 108). If this is not possible then correction of an acidosis must be empirical. As a rough guide, in a mild acidosis, there is likely to be a base deficit of 5 mmol/l; in severe cases it can be as much as 15 mmol/l or more.

It is wise to be cautious in the empirical administration of bicarbonate, however, for although an acidosis may be suspected from the history, it need not necessarily be present. It is always safer to err on the side of under-correction if in doubt. Excessive bicarbonate administration raises the blood pH (metabolic alkalosis) which results in respiratory depression and a shift in the haemoglobin dissociation curve, thus reducing the ability of haemoglobin to transfer oxygen to the tissues. Over-zealous correction of an acidosis will also shift potassium into the intracellular space and cause a hypokalaemia, as well as decreasing the concentration of ionized calcium in the blood which may precipitate hypocalcaemic tetany. In addition, too rapid an increase in arterial blood pH will be accompanied by a paradoxical fall in cerebrospinal fluid (CSF) pH as CSF bicarbonate levels lag behind plasma levels but CO_2 levels do not. This CSF acidosis causes a deterioration in cerebral function, respiratory disturbances and even tetany and convulsions. These considerations merely reinforce the desirability of laboratory data for monitoring acid—base disturbances.

A primary metabolic alkalosis, which may develop with severe vomiting, is treated by correcting the underlying cause, and restoring volume depletion by the administration of 0.9% saline. Specific acidifying agents are not required (Chapter 2).

Record keeping

It is vital to keep accurate and detailed records when treating any patient and fluid therapy is an area where good records can be invaluable in allowing the clinician to see immediately how the case is progressing. Ideally, a graphic form of monitoring vital signs such as temperature, pulse and respiration should be employed, together with

Fluid record

Daily req.	Date	Oral Time	Oral Type	Oral Total	Parenteral Type	Parenteral Start	Parenteral Finish	Total vol.	Urine	Vomit	Faeces	Insens loss	Output total
						Case No. vs 33339	Animal X Breed	Wt. 20 kg					
						Clinician AJW	Problem Pancreatitis	Maintenance Req. 1 litre					
1 litre	24/4/88	—	NIL	—	Hartmann's +	11.00 am	3pm	1 litre	✓	X	✓	N	
1 litre	25/4	9.00am ½ hrly	water 50ml @ a time	300ml	Hartmann's	2pm — 5pm	5pm	50D	✓	✓ 2x	✓	N	

Fig. 6.1 Sample fluid record chart.

a simple record of fluid input and output. An example of a simple fluid balance chart is shown in Fig. 6.1.

In addition to keeping a record chart it can also be useful to formulate a plan of action each day with regard to both the underlying disease problem and fluid requirements, and Fig. 6.2 summarizes a suitable plan to be followed for daily fluid requirements.

Case examples

Case example 1

The following case involving circumstances where the animal could not experience thirst nor control its intake illustrates the usefulness of the case history and emphasizes how an animal can build up a substantial fluid deficit when the intake is curtailed, in the absence of abnormal losses.

A 30 kg adult German Shepherd dog suffered cardiac arrest due to failure of the oxygen supply during a general anaesthetic. Apparently adequate cardiovascular and pulmonary function were restored by standard resuscitative procedures but the animal failed to regain consciousness. Fluid intake and spontaneous urine output in the following 2 days were nil. On the first day a diuretic was administered and 300 ml of urine were passed, but on the second day the urinary output was less than 20 ml. On the third day it was decided (belatedly) that the animal should be rehydrated.

The probable fluid deficit was considered to be mainly water depletion since there had been no losses in vomit or faeces and the

Summary
1 Calculate deficit
2 Estimate ongoing losses
3 Decide on type of fluid
4 Does it need $NaHCO_3$?
5 Does it need K^+?
6 Work out maintenance requirements
7 Add 1, 2 and 6, divide by hours
8 Convert 7 to drops/minute
9 Mark bag off in hours
10 Keep input/output chart

Fig. 6.2 Action plan for calculating fluid requirements.

probable extent of this depletion was calculated as 3 × 20 ml/kg inevitable loss (1.8 l) plus the urinary losses (320 ml), so that the animal was probably short of some 2.12 l of water. It was recognized that replacement of this deficit should take at least 24 hours and because there was no reason to suspect lack of renal concentrating capacity, a 24-hour maintenance allowance (40 ml/kg or 1.2 l) was added to this. From this calculation a total intake of 3.32 l of N/5 saline was prescribed for the third day (4.6 ml/kg/hour). During the latter part of this day the dog regained consciousness. It started to eat and drink and from then on fluid and food intake presented no problem. The animal recovered uneventfully.

Case example 2

A flat-coated Retriever (30 kg) was presented collapsed and moribund, 2 days after a road traffic accident. There was no vomiting. There was dysrhythmia (ectopics) until after 4 pm. Initially, acid–base data were not available but the hyperkalaemia demanded treatment — hence bicarbonate at 1.6 mmol/kg (correction of assumed acidosis — guideline 5, Table 6.4). The second dose of bicarbonate was calculated (deficit 15 mmol/l in 30/3 l, i.e. 150 mmol total deficit). Half correction (initial treatment) required 75 mmol. This case illustrates four aspects of dealing with hyperkalaemia and thereby restoring normal cardiac function prior to surgery:

1 Correction of acidosis.
2 Use of glucose.

Table 6.2 Case example 2, venous blood sample findings

	Admission (noon)	2 pm	4 pm	5 pm
pH	—	7.188	7.318	7.389
K mmol/l	7.1	4.7	4.0	
Urea mmol/l	40	26	18	
PCV %	44	38	33	
Base deficit mmol/l	—	15	8	3
			Peritoneal dialysis	
Treatment	2 litres N/5 saline + 4.3% glucose + 50 mmol bicarbonate (1.6 mmol/kg)		Repeat 2 litres glucose saline + 75 mmol bicarbonate, 10 ml Ca gluconate i.v.	

3 Use of calcium.
4 Peritoneal dialysis.
The uraemia was post-renal (ruptured bladder). This was successfully treated surgically at 5 pm, following correction of the major
disturbances.

Case example 3

A 3-year-old Labrador was presented collapsed with sustained
vomiting. Venous blood showed:

Urea	38
PCV	50
pH	7.451
Base deficit	−16

Again, uraemia but this time pre-renal, i.e. caused by the severe
dehydration (PCV = 50). Renal failure is unlikely to present with the
severe metabolic alkalosis seen in this animal (base deficit of *minus*
16, i.e. base excess). The problem was duodenal obstruction (rubber
ball) and it was corrected surgically after correction of volume depletion
by 'normal' saline (correction of metabolic alkalosis).

Case example 4

A 3-year-old King Charles Spaniel presented with profuse vomiting,
unable to stand and x-rays showed gas-filled loops of bowel. Venous
blood showed:

K	2.2
pH	7.428
Base deficit	−5

The striking feature was the hypokalaemia — and the radiographic
indication of ileus. It was treated with Hartmann's, to which 25 mmol/l
of K^+ was added (a total of 1 litre over 12 hours). Recovery occurred
within 12 hours, including cessation of both vomiting and ileus. The
rationale of using Hartmann's solution, despite the alkalosis, was that
the alkalosis was mild and likely to respond to volume replacement;
the crucial decision was to give K^+. A saline−KCl mixture could have
been used.

Case example 5

An 18-month-old Golden Retriever was presented collapsed following severe vomiting and general malaise. Venous blood showed:

pH	6.987
K	7.6
Base deficit	23.5

The key feature of this case is the severe acidosis and hyperkalaemia, despite the vomiting; blood urea was above 40 mmol/l. This was renal failure due to renal dysplasia and treatment was therefore inappropriate.

Case example 6

The following data were obtained from a collapsed and vomiting 6-year-old Springer Spaniel (18 kg):

	Before treatment	*After treatment*
pH	7.151	7.326
Base deficit	17	8.6
Urea	14	12
K	8.0	5.5
Na	128.1	131.0
PCV	54	50

The case was one of Addison's disease and the data indicate the severity of the acidosis and hyperkalaemia despite the profuse vomiting (Chapter 12). Treatment consisted of appropriate steroid therapy plus 0.9% saline, with added bicarbonate (50 mmol initially; a further 50 mmol after the second sample).

All the preceding cases illustrate the variety of disturbances associated with collapsed and vomiting dogs, and the importance of obtaining laboratory data wherever possible.

Table 6.3 Data showing that in the absence of diarrhoea, metabolic alkalosis is a common feature of gastrointestinal disturbances in ruminants (see Chapter 9)

	VI	RDA	LDA	LDA	I
pH	7.518	7.530	7.549	7.406	7.398
Base deficit	−26.5	−34.9	−21.3	−10.7	−3.9

Table 6.4 Safety guidelines

1 Deficits	50–150 ml/kg (5–15% of BWt)	
2 Correction	50% in first 6 hours 75% in 24 hours 100% in 48 hours — monitor progress	
3 Initial rates	10 ml/kg/hour gives 6% BWt in 6 hours (50% of 12% deficit) 15 ml/kg/hour gives 9% BWt in 6 hours (50% of 18% deficit!) Given in 1 hour, 9% BWt (90 ml/kg/hour) is a very *high* rate, normally needed only in shock and then not for too long	
4 K^+	Max. 0.5 mmol/kg/hour hence best to stay below 30 mmol/l (up to 15 ml/kg/hour)	
5 HCO_3^-		Replacing at 10 mmol/l of ECF corrects mild acidosis and converts severe to mild Pretend ECF is 33% BWt (allows for extra H^+ in cells too) and you need 3.3 mmol/kg BWt *But initially (as always for deficit therapy) give 50% estimated deficit (1.6 mmol/kg)*
6 Maintenance water		50 ml/kg/day *approximately* (variable!) *inevitable* loss 20 ml/kg/day (urine conserved)
7 Maintenance energy		50 kcal/kg/day *approximately* (variable!) 1 g glucose aq. = 3.4 kcal 0.5 g/kg/hour = max. rate to avoid urinary excretion of glucose
8 Colloids		Max. dose 20% blood volume, i.e. 20 ml/kg approx. to avoid possible clotting problems (especially dextrans)

1 kcal = 4.2 kJ.

Case example 7

The data given in Table 6.3 were obtained from a number of cows with vagal indigestion (VI), right displaced abomasum (RDA), left displaced abomasum (LDA) and intussusception (I).

Safety guidelines [11]

The primary aim of this book is to promote a rational rather than a 'rote' approach to fluid therapy. It is useful, however, to have in mind, in a wallet or on a wall, a few guidelines which will make the initial treatment reasonably appropriate in magnitude and rate, and almost certainly safe. Table 6.4 should serve this purpose.

References

1 Hall, L.W. (1967) *Fluid Balance in Canine Surgery*, 90−9. Bailliere, London.
2 Waterman, A.E. (1984) Disorders of fluid and electrolyte balance. In: *Canine Medicine and Therapeutics* (2nd edn), 316−39. Chandler, E.A., Sutton, J.B. & Thompson, D.J. (eds). Blackwell Scientific Publications, Oxford.
3 Cornelius, L.M. (1980) Fluid therapy in small animal practice. *Journal of the American Veterinary Medical Association* **176**, 10−17.
4 Groutides, C.P. (1988) Studies of fluid, electrolyte and acid−base balance in diarrhoeic calves with special reference to fluid therapy. PhD Thesis, University of London.
5 Michell, A.R. (1979) The physiological basis of fluid therapy in small animals. *Veterinary Record* **104**, 542−8.
6 Cornelius, L.M., Finco D.R. & Culver, D.H. (1978) Physiological effects of rapid infusion of Ringer's lactate solution into dogs. *American Journal of Veterinary Research* **39**, 1185−90.
7 Haskins, S.C. (1983) Shock. In: *Current Veterinary Therapy VIII*, 2−27. Kirk, R.W. (ed). W.B. Saunders, Philadelphia.
8 Kitchell, B.F. & Haskins, S.C. (1984) Feline trauma and critical care medicine. *Veterinary Clinics of North America: Small Animal Practice* **14**, 1331−44.
9 Boothe, H.W., Clark, D.R. & Merton, D.A. (1985) Cardiovascular effects of rapid infusion of crystalloid in the hypovolaemic cat. *Journal of Small Animal Practice* **26**, 477−89.
10 Muylle, E., Van den Hende, C., Nuytten, J., Deprez, P., Vlaminck, K. & Oyaert, W. (1984) Potassium concentration in equine red blood cells. *Equine Veterinary Journal* **16**, 447−52.
11 Michell, A.R. (1983) Understanding fluid therapy. *Irish Veterinary Journal* **37**, 94−103.

Chapter 7
Routes and techniques of fluid administration

Routes of fluid administration

Fluid therapy may be administered by the following routes:
1 Alimentary — oral and rectal.
2 Subcutaneous.
3 Intraperitoneal.
4 Intravenous.

The alimentary route of fluid administration has many major advantages. The fluids need not be sterile, nor need the composition be absolutely what is required as selective absorption occurs. As a result, large volumes may be given inexpensively. However, for this route to be effective, the alimentary system must remain capable of absorption, and this route therefore cannot be used in cases of extensive vomiting, or in circulatory shock. Although most alimentary fluid therapy is given via the oral route, fluid is absorbed from the large intestine, so in theory the rectal route of administration can also be used, for example in piglets.

The subcutaneous route requires fluids which are sterile, isotonic and non-irritant. Ideally, they should have similar electrolyte composition to normal plasma since 'missing' ions may be drawn out of circulation until the subcutaneous pool is absorbed. Absorption depends on adequate circulation, so that this route is of no use once circulatory insufficiency is present as vasoconstriction of the subcutaneous vessels occurs early in the process of shock. In particular, the subcutaneous route should never be used where cardiovascular collapse has made venous catheterization difficult to perform. Sterility is essential, as infection occurs easily. The volumes that can be given are small and absorption limited, so the route is really only practicable for the administration of ionic solutions for maintenance in animals already reasonably well hydrated.

The intraperitoneal route also requires fluids which are sterile, non-irritant and isotonic. However, considerably larger volumes may be administered, and the very large area for absorption and the fact that blood vessels to this area are constricted later in the course of circulatory failure means that the method may still be of use in cases where some fluid deficit already exists. The solutions should be close to body temperature both for comfort and maximal absorption.

The intravenous route is the only satisfactory route when rapid rehydration of the animal is required, e.g. in circulatory shock, as it is the only route where the fluid is placed directly into the circulation. Indeed, it is the only route by which parenteral nutrition, blood products and blood substitutes may be given. This immediate entry to the circulatory system carries with it, however, the risk of circulatory overload through over-transfusion, particularly if the fluid being administered cannot be removed from the circulation either by redistribution through the body compartments, or by renal excretion. Fluids for intravenous administration must ideally be sterile and pyrogen-free, and isotonic in order not to cause haemolysis or to irritate the vessel wall.

Presentation of commercially available fluids

Fluids purchased commercially usually come supplied in the following:
1 Glass bottles.
2 Semi-rigid plastic containers.
3 Soft plastic bags (plasticized polyvinyl chloride) (Fig. 7.1).

Where bottles are used, it is necessary to let air into the bottle in order for the fluid to come out. This is done either by an air inlet on the drip set (Fig. 7.2), the use of a flutter valve (Fig. 7.3), or placing a needle into the bottle. The disadvantage in this system is the loss of sterility, and the danger that when the drip runs out, air will be drawn into the veins. In order to ensure that this does not happen, if practicable, the tubing from the drip set should dip well below the level of the animal before it reaches the intravenous catheter, and the animal should remain under constant supervision.

The majority of purchased fluids come in soft plastic bags. These, used with a fluid-giving set (which is sometimes provided as an integral part of the set), empty completely, without allowing any air

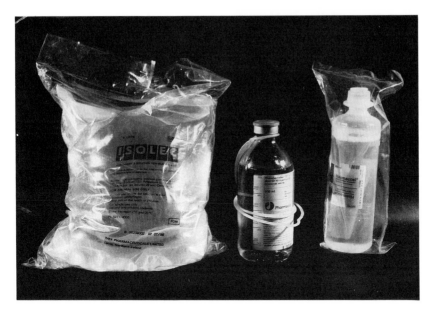

Fig. 7.1 Containers with commercially prepared fluids.

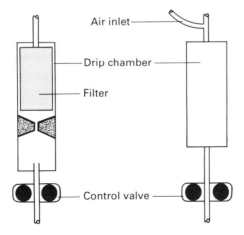

Fig. 7.2 Drip chambers with filter (left) for blood or blood products, air inlet (right) for rigid bottles.

in the system, thus ensuring sterility, and removing the risk of air embolus.

Some fluids (e.g. Haemaccel, the Polyfusor range) come in stiff plastic bottles. Although the bottles collapse to some extent as they

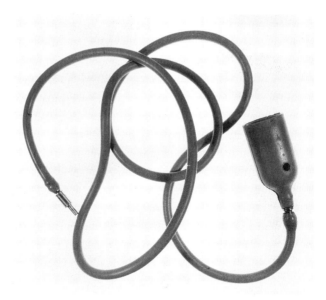

Fig. 7.3 Flutter valve.

empty, and most of the fluid will leave without resort to an air inlet, their use in this way does result in considerable wastage. If air is allowed in to reduce this wastage, then the system suffers from the same disadvantages as the glass bottles.

Fluid administration sets

Fluid administration sets all have a drip chamber. Those used for the administration of blood or blood products require an efficient filter (Fig. 7.2). The sets may or may not have an air inlet blanked off, but available if required for use with a non-collapsible bottle. In use, the drip chamber should be primed to be about half-full, so as to prevent the entrapment of air, and to allow the speed of flow of fluid through the drip chamber to be observed. The administration set may be extended if required by the use of a drip extension set.

Micro-drip sets (Fig. 7.4) are available for use in cases where it is essential to know accurately the volume of fluid given. They consist of a 100 ml chamber with attached fluid administration set. By prefilling the chamber with a limited amount of fluid, the danger of inadvertent over-administration is avoided. These sets are essential when fluids

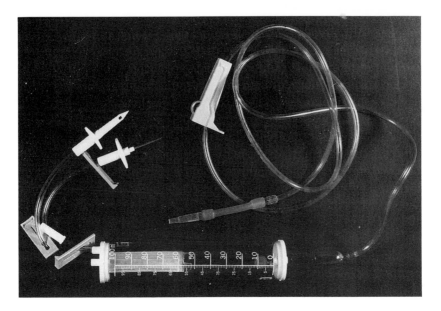

Fig. 7.4 'Micro' administration set for small volume.

which will remain in the circulation (e.g. blood, blood products) are given to very small animals.

Temperature control

Fluids given by the intravenous, subcutaneous or intraperitoneal routes should be warmed to blood temperature before administration in order to prevent hypothermia, and if large volumes are given orally, it is still advantageous to warm them first. The most accurate method of heating fluids for intravenous use is to pass them through a blood warming coil (Chapter 8) which is either encased in a thermostatically controlled heating unit, or, more simply, immersed in a thermostatically controlled water bath. Failing these, the blood warming coil may be immersed in a bowl of warm water, but where thermostatic controls are not used great care must be taken *not to overheat* the fluid. The packs of fluid should be prewarmed, but unless administration is fast, significant cooling still occurs in the drip tubing. Where methods of reheating the fluid in the drip tubing are not available (such as in the field situation with large animals), then loss of heat may be limited by covering the fluid container and drip tubing with some form of lagging. Enclosing the apparatus in containers of polystyrene beads provides a practical method of achieving this end.

Techniques of intravenous fluid administration

Fluids may be administered intravenously by means of:
1 Needles.
2 Catheters placed in the vein through a needle.
3 Catheters placed in the vein over a needle.

Needles

All intravenous needles, although comparatively inexpensive and easy to place, suffer the disadvantage that they are easily dislodged from or through the vein. Needles for intravenous administration are now made with a variety of 'side wings' to help anchor them in position. The commonest version of these is the 'butterfly' (Fig. 7.5) which also has an attached length of light plastic tubing to enable injections to be

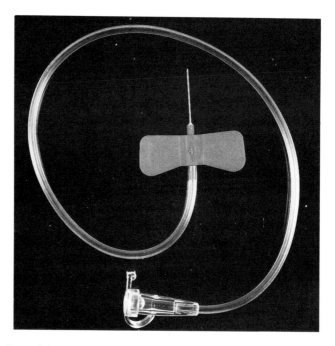

Fig. 7.5 'Butterfly' type winged needle.

made without disturbing the needle. However, even with such adaptations, needles are of no use for the administration of large volumes of fluid, and are difficult to keep patent in the ambulant patient.

Catheters through a needle

If a large-bore needle is placed in a vein, a catheter may be placed through it, advanced well into the vein, then the needle withdrawn (Fig. 7.6). This method of placing a catheter is extremely dangerous as there is always the chance that the catheter may become cut off at the bevel of the needle, leaving a length of plastic free in the circulation. A much safer variation of this method is the 'Seldinger technique' in which a wire is placed through the intravenous needle, the needle withdrawn, then the catheter slid over the wire into the vein. The safest and simplest adaptation of the method is to replace

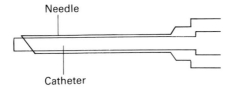

Fig. 7.6 Catheter through needle.

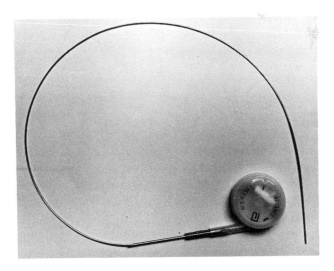

Fig. 7.7 Commercial long catheter through catheter ('Drum Reel': Abbott Laboratories).

the original intravenous needle with a wide but short catheter. A longer, narrower catheter may then be placed through this. This 'catheter through catheter' method is utilized for placing very long catheters, such as the Abbott drum reel (Fig. 7.7).

Catheter over a needle (Figure 7.8)

These are the most useful method of intravenous cannulation. The catheter consists of a plastic sheath over a slightly longer needle, the end of which is made of clear plastic, the 'flash chamber', so that when the vein is penetrated, the flow back of blood can be seen. A plug prevents blood from escaping. Catheters of this type are available in a wide range of lengths and diameters (Fig. 7.9). Figure 7.10 a–f illustrates the method of inserting a catheter into a vessel. Sometimes, particularly if a wide-bore catheter is being used, it is necessary first to make a small hole in the skin. The needle and catheter unit are inserted into the vein (Fig. 7.10b) and blood will be seen in the flash

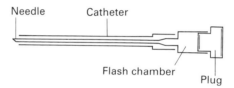

Fig. 7.8 Catheter over needle.

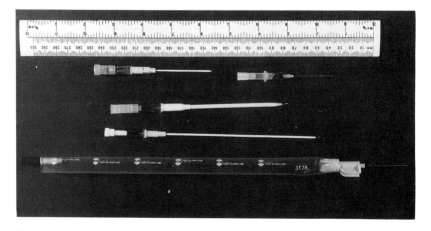

Fig. 7.9 A range of commercially available 'over the needle' catheters.

chamber. The plastic catheter is then advanced further into the blood vessel, leaving the needle exactly where it is (Fig. 7.10c, d). Once the catheter is inserted to its hilt, the needle is withdrawn (Fig. 7.10e), the drip attached, and the catheter is anchored in place. The reason for placing the catheter in this way is that if, once the catheter unit is in the vein, the whole unit is advanced, it may penetrate the further side of the vessel. If the needle is partially withdrawn before advancing the plastic catheter, the catheter often fails to slide up the vein. Once the needle has been partly withdrawn, it must not be reinserted into the catheter, otherwise the needle may penetrate the side of the catheter, causing the tip of the catheter to break.

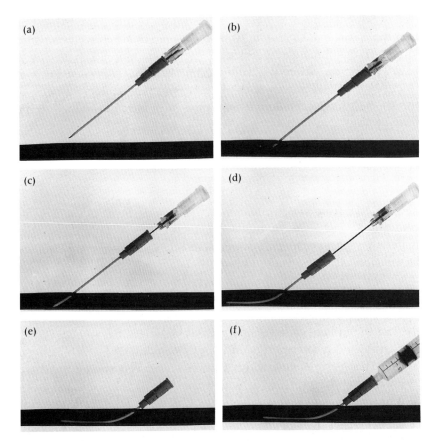

Fig. 7.10 (a–f) Diagram of placement of 'over the needle' catheter into a vein; (a–b) Catheter assembly placed in vein; (c–d) Plastic catheter is advanced, leaving the needle exactly where it is; (e) Needle is withdrawn; (f) Syringe is attached.

The E–Z Cath (Fig. 7.9) is a variation of the catheter over needle, designed to place very long catheters into the vessels. In this case the needle continues as a wire, and the whole unit is packed in a plastic sleeve in such a way that the catheter may be put in place without being touched by the operator.

Choice of catheter

There is now a wide range of different makes, materials, diameters and lengths of intravenous catheters available commercially. The size and length of catheter selected will mainly be governed by the species, size of patient, speed of fluid administration required, and the time that the catheter is to remain in place. Where fluid replacement is for long term maintenance, then long catheters are more likely to stay in place. However, where rapid fluid administration is needed, such as in circulatory collapse, then the largest possible diameter catheter of the shortest practicable length will present minimal resistance to the flow of fluid.

Flow characteristics of catheters can be represented by

$$\text{Flow} = \frac{\text{K (a constant)} \times \text{diameter}^4 \times \text{pressure gradient}}{\text{length} \times \text{viscosity}}$$

The material from which the catheter is manufactured influences the constant K, but as most modern catheters are of teflon, or other materials with excellent flow characteristics, it is rarely the limiting factor clinically. The most important factor is the diameter of the tube, and it is essential that catheters of an adequate diameter are used where the fluid has to be administered quickly. However, increased length is also important in causing increased resistance, and the fact that a long catheter is less easily dislodged has to be weighed against the increased resistance to flow when deciding which catheter to use. The speed of flow through the catheter can also be increased by increasing the pressure at which the fluid is infused, such as by raising the height above the patient of a bag of fluid, or by putting positive pressure on the bag of fluid, for example, with a pressure infusor bag (Fig. 7.11). However, positive pressure should only be applied to systems where no air can gain access to the circuit, otherwise the danger of air embolism is high should the drip fluid run out.

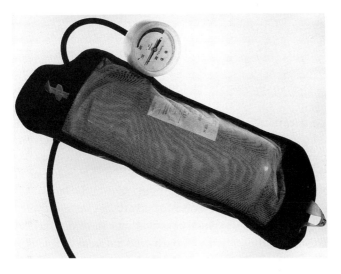

Fig. 7.11 Bag for infusing fluids under pressure (Travenol Laboratories).

Once the length and diameter of catheter has been decided, further choice from the huge range of excellent products available is a matter of personal preference and they are constantly being revised. Nevertheless, some details of design are worth noting. In all well manufactured catheters the plastic catheter is closely applied to the inserting needle, as any 'step' between the two makes insertion difficult. In large diameter catheters it is usually necessary for the catheter edge to be bevelled, and in the largest diameter catheters (such as the 10 G Angiocath, Deseret) the inserting needle has an outer coating to ensure there is no such 'step' (Fig. 7.9). The majority of catheters are sufficiently flexible to prevent damage to the veins, but adequately rigid to allow easy insertion into veins or arteries; however in some species (in the authors' experience notably sheep) such catheters tend to penetrate through the vein; in these cases the more flexible catheters, such as the Cathlon IV (Critikon) may be preferable. Another point to consider is the attachment of the catheter to the hub. Usually a straight catheter is attached to a hub of different material. These catheters are easy to insert and to keep in the vein, but may kink at the point of attachment to the hub. Some catheters (e.g. Braunule) have no join, the catheter gradually widening to become the hub (Fig. 7.9). Such catheters are less likely to kink, but tend to slide out of the vein unless very well anchored into place.

Maintenance of catheters

All intravenous catheters should be placed into the veins using aseptic techniques. Asepsis is absolutely essential if the catheter is to be left in place, as the small blood or fibrin clots which form around the catheter provide an ideal medium for bacterial growth.

Where a catheter is to be left in place whilst not in use, some method of preventing blood from filling the catheter and from clotting must be employed. For most types of catheters it is possible to purchase plastic stillettes which are pushed down the catheter, keeping it patent and empty of blood until next required (Fig. 7.12). Other methods involve sealing the end of the catheter with a three-way tap or a rubber seal through which it is possible to inject (Fig. 7.12) and then filling the catheter with heparinized saline.

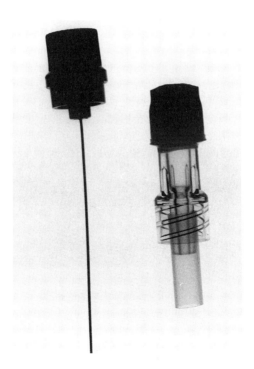

Fig. 7.12 Methods for preventing blood from clotting in a catheter: stillette (left) or rubber cap (right) through which heparinized saline can be injected.

Species detail

Dog and cat [1]

Oral administration

In the conscious dog, oral fluid therapy is best taken voluntarily by mouth. Otherwise, when necessary, the skin fold at the side of the mouth is tensed, and fluid gently poured in from a spoon or syringe; the head is then tilted up, and the dog's throat massaged until it swallows. To avoid inhalation of fluid, care must be taken to keep quantities small and to give the dog plenty of time to swallow. If oral hydration using the mouth is not possible, for example due to jaw or oesophageal lesions, then a pharyngostomy tube may be used (Fig. 7.13). Once put in place under anaesthesia, these tubes are well tolerated by the conscious animal and may be left in place for several days, allowing fluid and liquidized food to be administered. Silicon tubing is ideal as it is non-irritant and does not often kink or obstruct. Whenever such a tube is left in place it must be carefully checked before every use in order to ensure that it is still in the alimentary tract as it is possible for the tube to be regurgitated and inhaled. Also, before the introduction of any fluid through the tube, an attempt must be made to aspirate fluid from the stomach, as there is no point in giving fluid if ileus is present and fluids are accumulating in the gastrointestinal tract.

The major difference in treatment of the cat from the dog is due to temperament, and to the fact that cats resent restraint and handling. Oral dosing of cats must be handled with care and tact; they will usually accept oral fluid administered from a small syringe (Fig. 7.14). In our experience, cats tolerate pharyngostomy tubes very well, and their use should always be considered if oral hydration is likely to be necessary for several days.

Intravenous administration

Although many veterinary surgeons use the cephalic vein for intravenous therapy, the jugular vein is the route of choice in the dog and it is essential for parenteral nutrition (Chapter 12). It is large, accessible, and in most cases (excluding the very fat dog) it is extremely easy to catheterize percutaneously, after a small skin incision has been made. Most veterinary surgeons prefer to restrain the dog on its side, and

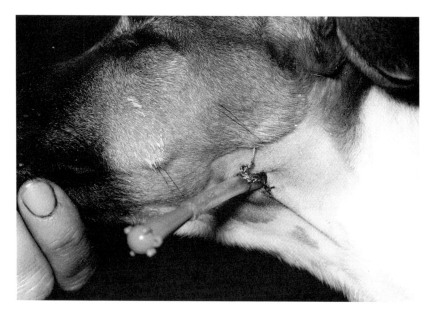

Fig. 7.13 Pharyngostomy tube in a dog.

direct the tip of the catheter towards the heart (Fig. 7.15). The advantages of the use of the jugular are that it allows an adequate diameter of catheter to be used, permitting the rapid administration of large quantities of fluid, long catheters can be passed into the right atrium if required, and accurate measurements of central venous or right atrial pressure can be obtained. Because of the amount of skin mobility, a fairly long catheter is essential. A 2–3 inch (5–7.5 cm) catheter, although possibly adequate in a collapsed or anaesthetized patient, is too short for the mobile animal, and the longer (e.g. 5.25 inch; Angiocath, Deseret) catheters, or the even longer E–Z caths (Deseret) should be employed. The catheter should be sutured in place, and the attached drip tubing sutured or bandaged as shown in Fig. 7.22 so that if the dog pulls on the drip, the drip tube kinks rather than the catheter becoming displaced. It is an advantage to have the drip suspended by a spring, or to use a spring-shaped drip extension tube (e.g. Vygon), which again allows the dog greater mobility.

If the dog is in such a state of cardiovascular collapse that percutaneous catheterization is impossible, then it is necessary to cut down to expose the vein for catheterization. The dog is restrained on its side with its neck elevated over a sandbag or cotton wool, its neck

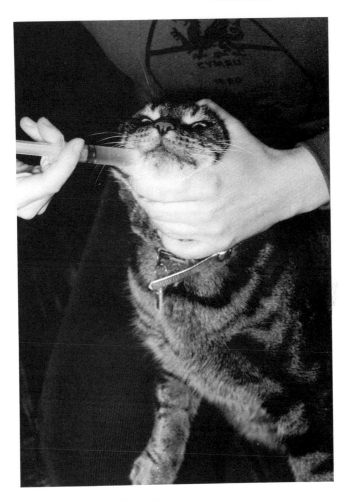

Fig. 7.14 Cat restrained for oral fluid administration.

is clipped and cleaned (aseptic precautions are essential) and local anaesthetic infiltrated into the skin. The surgeon then cuts through the skin, subcutaneous tissue, and cutaneous muscle until the vein is exposed. Often if such a cut down has been necessary the vein, when found, consists of a thin, blue, thread-like structure, and it is obvious why it was not initially palpable. A piece of suture material is placed under the vein so it can be elevated; this allows the blood to collect anteriorly, distending the vein and usually making insertion of the catheter easy. Sometimes it is necessary to make a small cut in the vein, hold the edge of the vein with fine forceps, and insert the

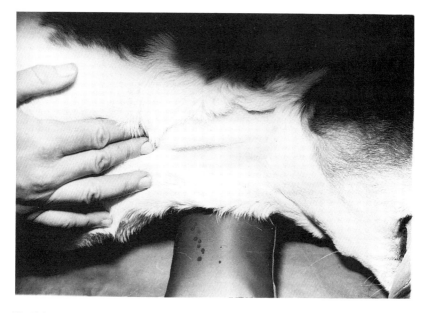

Fig. 7.15 Jugular vein raised for catheterization in a dog.

catheter in this way. When the tip of the catheter is in the vein, the vein is easily distensible and it is possible to use a large-bore catheter. It must be emphasized that it is precisely in such cases, where cardiovascular collapse prevents easy catheterization, that *it is essential for the animal to receive rapid fluid replacement by the intravenous route*, and that a large-bore jugular catheter is the only method by which this can be done at adequate speed.

For short term therapy in animals not requiring rapid fluid administration, the cephalic and tarsal veins are simple and quick sites to catheterize. An adequate diameter of catheter should always be employed. An 18 G catheter can easily be inserted into the cephalic vein of all but the tiniest dogs. As the skin is less mobile than over the jugular vein, a 2–3 inch catheter is usually an adequate length, indeed longer ones tend to kink as they go around the bend of the elbow. Catheters and drip tubing should be anchored by tape or sutures around the leg, incorporating a loop of drip tubing in an S-bend. Again, attachment in this way, and attachment of the drip bag to a spring of some sort allows the animal considerable movement, without resulting in dislodgement of the catheter.

In the conscious unshocked cat, jugular catheterization can be difficult, as the cat resents the restraint necessary; heavy sedation or anaesthesia may be required. Indeed, if the cat is anaesthetized for surgery, this is the time to consider its future fluid requirements, thus avoiding further anaesthesia for catheterization. If the cat is severely dehydrated and shocked, however, restraint is no problem. The method of jugular catheterization is the same in the cat as for the dog. There is considerable skin mobility over the jugular vein, so a 5–6 inch catheter, although it seems long, is usually necessary if it is to remain in place in the mobile animal. Again in the cat, cephalic and tarsal veins may be used. It should be possible to insert an 18 G catheter into the cephalic vein of an adult cat. If the catheter is to remain *in situ* in a mobile cat, then it must be particularly well anchored in place and protected by bandages to prevent the cat from removing it. In general, however, sick cats tolerate intravenous catheters remarkably well, and in our experience attempts by the cat to remove the catheter usually indicate the presence of infection or pain.

In small animals there is a particular danger of overloading the animal with fluid and causing oedema. Regular monitoring of central venous pressure should reduce the risk. However, it is safest to limit the amount of fluid which can be given at any time by devices such as the mini-drip set already described. Infusion pumps are ideal but very expensive. The correct temperature of fluid administration is particularly important in small animals, as hypothermia is easily induced.

Large animals

Oral administration

Although horses and cattle may be drenched by holding the head up and tipping fluid into the mouth from a bottle, this method usually results in fluid everywhere except in the animal. Stomach tubing is simple to perform and is the method of choice for oral administration of fluids to large animals. In the horse, a smooth and well lubricated stomach tube is passed through the ventral nasal meatus. The smooth edge and lubrication are essential as they reduce the risk of nasal haemorrhage. Even a well-sedated horse will usually throw its head in the air as the tube is first inserted into its nose and the tube should be held firmly to the nostril (Fig. 7.16) so that it is not dislodged at

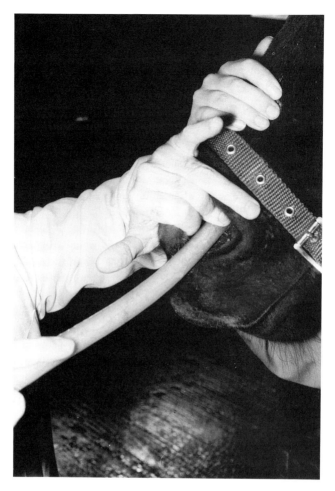

Fig. 7.16 Insertion of stomach tube into the horse's nostril (note method of anchoring tube).

this time. The horse usually tolerates passage of the tube fairly well once it is through the nasal meatus. As the tube reaches the pharynx, it is necessary to make the horse swallow (jiggling the tube helps) to make the tube pass into the oesophagus rather than the trachea. It is in fact extremely difficult to pass a stomach tube in the anaesthetized horse, and even deep sedation which reduces the swallowing reflexes tends to encourage the tube to pass down the trachea. As the natural line is nasal cavity to trachea (the horse is a nose breather), it may take several attempts to ensure the tube is in the correct passage. If the tube is in the oesophagus it should be possible to palpate it on the left side of the neck, whilst it cannot be palpated if in the trachea. If the stomach tube is in the trachea it should be possible to feel air movement from the tube as the horse exhales (Fig. 7.17); however if a small stomach tube, or one with side holes is employed, this air movement is slight, and is best detected by holding the end of the tube to the operator's face. As the consequences of placing fluid in the trachea instead of the oesophagus are disastrous, great care must be taken to ensure the stomach tube is correctly placed before any fluid is administered. Once it is certain the tube is in the oesophagus it should be advanced to the stomach; at this stage, stomach gases may be released.

Horse stomach tubes are manufactured in red rubber, silicone rubber or in plastic, and may have end or side holes. Plastic tubes tend to be too stiff when cold, and may need warming to soften before use. The silicone tubes have the advantage that their flexibility is not altered by temperature, but these tubes must be well lubricated as otherwise they do not pass easily through the nasal passages. When the purpose of the stomach tube is to give fluid, then as long as the tube has been pushed far enough to reach the stomach, it is

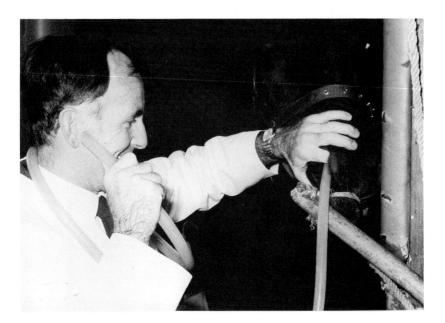

Fig. 7.17 Checking that the stomach tube is correctly placed.

immaterial whether the tube has end or side holes. If the tube is in the oesophagus, however, an end hole is preferable as the side holes may become blocked by the oesophageal wall. If the tube is being used to ensure that the stomach does not already contain food or fluid (as it will in cases of intestinal obstruction or of paralytic ileus) then an end hole is less likely to become blocked.

At the end of the procedure the stomach tube should be withdrawn as carefully and steadily as possible. Unfortunately, at this stage the horse again often throws up its head, and the subsequent pull on the tube may cause profuse nasal haemorrhage from damaged turbinate structures.

For long term fluid administration, the stomach tube may be left in place, and secured to a headcollar. However, in the authors' experience the tube is frequently displaced from the oesophagus to the trachea, so it is essential to check its situation before every fluid administration.

Oral rehydration fluids are frequently taken voluntarily by calves and, if not, stomach tubing is relatively simple. In adult cattle, stomach tubes are placed via the mouth rather than the nose (Figs 7.18−7.20). A drinkwater gag is placed between the molar teeth (Fig. 7.19). It is helpful to guide the stomach tube over the dorsum of the tongue by hand (Fig. 7.20), but once past this obstruction the tube usually passes easily into the oesophagus, and can then be advanced to the stomach. The correct positioning of the tube must be checked, as in the horse. As the stomach tube passes through the mouth, it tends to

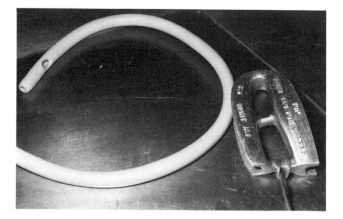

Fig. 7.18 Gag and stomach tube for cattle.

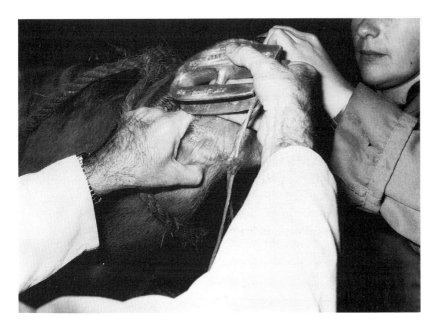

Fig. 7.19 Inserting the gag.

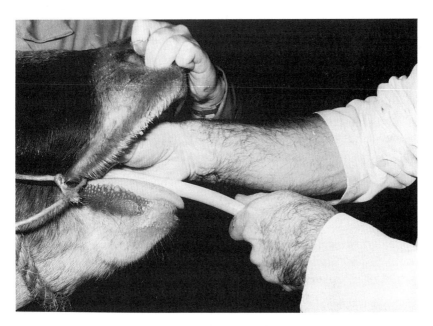

Fig. 7.20 Passing the stomach tube over the dorsum of the tongue.

become damaged by the rough teeth edges. Such roughened tubes should then be kept solely for use in cattle, as their subsequent use in a horse will frequently cause a nasal haemorrhage.

As ruminants come to be used more frequently as experimental animals, there is sometimes the need for long term fluid maintenance. In these situations, the presence of a ruminal cannula allows unlimited fluid to be placed straight into the rumen.

Fluids are absorbed from the large intestine, and in both ruminants and horses it is technically possible to administer fluids per rectum and have a significant proportion absorbed. Although this route is worth trying where all else fails, practically it is found that fluid administration results in straining, and that the majority is expelled before significant absorption has occurred.

Intravenous administration

The jugular vein is the most convenient and accessible vessel for catheterization in large animals. In these species the quantities of fluid which need to be given rapidly may be very large indeed, and if so then the greatest diameter catheter possible should be used. In the UK this is currently 10 G (Angiocath, Deseret), although larger catheters are available elsewhere. When using such large catheters it is always necessary to make a small skin incision (through a bleb of local anaesthetic), as the plastic will not slide easily through the skin. In the horse [2] there is limited skin mobility over the jugular vein and a 3 inch catheter will usually suffice, but in cattle, as the skin is more mobile, longer catheters are more likely to remain in place in the ambulatory animal. There is no easy alternative to the jugular vein in these species. Although the milk vein is sometimes used in cattle, the potential results of thrombosis or infection in this site make its use one of last resort. In horses, the external thoracic or limb veins have been used.

There are many practical problems related to the administration of i.v. fluid therapy in large animals. Firstly, the plastic bags of fluid available for use in man are generally too small. However, 3 and 5 l packs of some fluids are now commercially available as is the means to administer several of these bags simultaneously (Fig. 7.21). In the absence of these commercially available systems, suitable plastic containers may be used as reservoirs [3, 4].

Secondly, a collapsed animal suffering from dehydration amount-

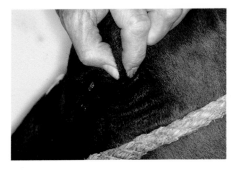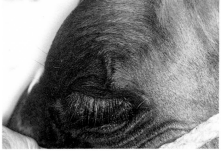

Plate 1 Decreased skin elasticity shown by 'tenting' after pinching eyelid (calf).

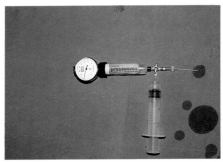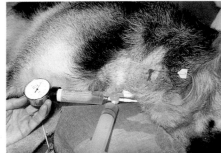

Plate 2 Aneroid system for measuring CVP.

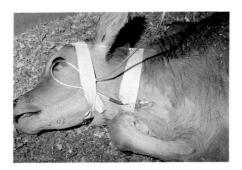

Plate 3 Method of anchoring the drip tubing in a calf — note the S-bend in the tube. (Sutures provide more secure anchorage than tape.)

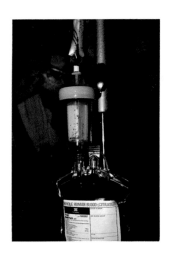

Plate 4 Blood filter.

[*facing page 142*]

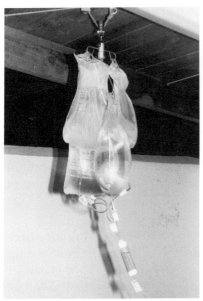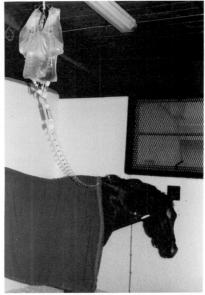

Fig. 7.21 Commercial fluid administration set for large volumes ('Stat i.v. set') (TMS Consultants, Yeovil).

ing to about 10% of its body weight will suffer haemoconcentration and hypotension and the effect of these changes will be to reduce venous return, thus making identification and cannulation of the jugular vein much more difficult than in a healthy animal. This, added to the lighting conditions often found on farms, accounts at least in part for the frequent frustration experienced by practitioners attempting the intravenous administration of fluids.

The difficulty in cannulation of the jugular vein in a collapsed animal can be reduced by lowering the animal's head or raising its hindquarters if convenient. In either case, the effect is to raise the pressure in the jugular vein, which then becomes more apparent and easier to cannulate successfully. In the case of a collapsed calf, this can be achieved by having the calf suspended with its hind legs over the pen gate, or, less dramatically, by lifting the calf onto a straw bale, and allowing the head to lie lower than the body. Having identified the jugular vein, it is often desirable to incise the skin over the site to assist the insertion of a cannula. This is especially necessary where the cannula used is designed to insert into the vein over the needle, since these are very difficult to pass through the skin of a calf, which is both thick and tough. The skin is held in a pinch over the vein, and an incision is made over and parallel to the vein. In this way, insertion of the needle with the cannula is relatively straightforward.

There is a temptation to use a rigid needle rather than a cannula for fluid administration to a collapsed animal. This frequently results from the lack of a suitable sheathed cannula, or from the slightly increased difficulty in inserting such a cannula in comparison with a needle. However, the use of a cannula gives the opportunity for prolonged administration over hours or days, while a needle is only suitable for use over a short period, and even then any movement of the patient is likely to dislodge the needle from the vein. So, wherever possible, a suitable cannula should be used, and after insertion should be held in position by a suture through the skin.

In order to increase the pressure of administration of fluids, either the reservoir may be placed well above the height of the animal, thus utilizing gravity as is generally done in small animals, or the container may be pressurized by pumping air into it. This latter approach does run the risk of serious air embolism occurring should the reservoir run out of fluid. If large amounts of fluid are given quickly, then the drip administration tubing must be of wide diameter. A commercial set for the administration of large volumes of fluid is shown in Fig. 7.21, and a suitable 'home-made' apparatus well described by Corke [3].

It may be necessary to continue fluid administration for several days. Where it is necessary to continue parenteral fluids for some time in the ambulatory animal, the principles are as those described for the small animal. In these circumstances, catheters must be of an adequate length and sutured into place. The attached drip tubing may be bandaged or sutured to the neck, with a loop of tubing ensuring that pull on the set does not remove the catheter (Plate 3). Methods of fixing the tubing further depend on the restraint of the animal, but as described before, the use of a spring, rubber bands or of a spiral drip tube, does allow the animal considerable freedom of movement (Fig. 7.22).

Preparation of fluids for i.v. use

For small animals there is no reason to use anything but commercially available fluids which are sterile and pyrogen-free, but for large animals the quantities required may be so great that veterinary surgeons

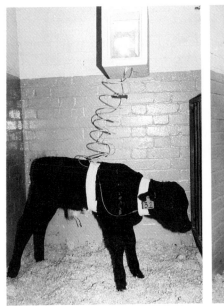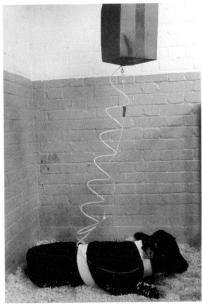

Fig. 7.22 Spiral drip tubing allowing the calf freedom of movement. (Used in this case to support conventional tubing. Note the polystyrene insulation.)

may consider making the fluids themselves. It must be stressed that the preparation of such fluids requires immaculate attention to detail, as any fault in their make-up could result in the death of the patient.

Preparation of sterile, pyrogen-free water

The starting point for a practice-produced fluid must be a source of sterile water. Simple boiling does not, unfortunately, remove pyrogens. A straightforward technique for the preparation of sterile, pyrogen-free water 'in-house' has been described by Corke [3]. Tap water for human consumption in the UK should conform to standards laid down by the Council of European Communities (1980). This permits water containing a maximum total bacterial count of 100 organisms/ml to be supplied for human consumption. It should be emphasized that these are not permitted to include pathogenic species such as staphylococci, salmonellae or other coliforms. The non-pathogenic organisms in such water could nonetheless represent a severe challenge to the reticuloendothelial system if administered intravenously to an already debilitated patient. Tap water may also contain pyrogens in the form of lipopolysaccharide or lipoprotein derived from bacterial degradation.

Removal of bacteria and pyrogens from tap water may be achieved by distillation using a glass, quartz or suitable metal still, with a trap or baffle to remove droplets, which may otherwise enter the distillate and lead to contamination. A new or used still may be purchased, or it may be possible to obtain freshly distilled water from an institution possessing a suitable still. Distilled water tends to be quite acid due to dissolved gases, principally carbon dioxide, but the buffering capacity required to neutralize this is very small, so this acidity does not present a clinical problem even in acidotic patients. Stills are subject to inspection by H.M. Customs and Excise!

Ultrafiltration is another method of removing bacteria and pyrogens using a cellulose acetate filter of the Millipore type (Millipore (UK) Ltd) with a pore size of 0.22 μm or less. It is necessary to apply pressure across the filter to achieve sufficient flow rate. This may be done by using the commercial pressure filtering system manufactured by Millipore (UK) Ltd, or less expensively by applying suction to the receiving bottle whilst using a suitable filter funnel. Suction may be developed by using a mechanical air pump or a water vacuum pump. Filtration of a large volume requires a large diameter filter to prevent rapid clogging of the pores, and to obtain a satisfactory filtration rate.

Ultrafiltration, unlike distillation, does not affect the ionic composition of the purified water, but this is unlikely to cause a clinical problem. Even in hard water areas, the levels of calcium and magnesium are unlikely to exceed 2−3 mmol/l which are tolerable in intravenous fluids providing that this is allowed for whilst formulating the ionic composition. Local levels of ions in tap water should be obtained by reference to the local Water Board before developing a tap water-based system.

Preparation of solutions for correction of dehydration, acidosis or alkalosis

Hartmann's solution may conveniently be prepared in 20 litre aliquots by making up a concentrated solution of sodium, potassium and calcium chlorides in 1 litre of sterile water, which is then sterilized by autoclave. This concentrate, together with a measured quantity of autoclave-sterilized sodium lactate syrup, is diluted with 19 litres sterile water when required (Table 7.1).

Table 7.1 Hartmann's solution

Ionic composition of Hartmann's solution	
Sodium	130 mmol/l
Potassium	4 mmol/l
Calcium	2 mmol/l
Chloride	111 mmol/l
Lactate	27 mmol/l
Total	274 mmol of ions ≡ 274 mOsm/l (isotonic with plasma)

Preparation of Hartmann's solution
1 Prepare concentrated chloride solution (solution 1)

Sodium chloride	120 g
Potassium chloride	6 g
Calcium chloride (dihydrate)	5.83 g

Make up in 1 l of sterile water
Sterilize at 15 psi for 15 minutes

2 Prepare sodium lactate solution (solution 2)

Sodium lactate	85.6 ml of 70% syrup

Sterilize at 10 psi for 15 minutes

3 Add to solutions 1 and 2, 19 l of sterile water when needed

Modification of Hartmann's solution for metabolic alkalosis
1 Prepare concentrated chloride solution as in 1 above
2 Glucose 50% solution 400 ml (Boots Company, Nottingham)
3 Add to solutions 1 and 2, 19 l of sterile water
N.B   It may be desirable to add more potassium to the solution in the form of strong potassium chloride solution (Evans Medical, Dunstable, Beds)

Animals which are severely acidotic as well as being dehydrated may require more base than is present in the Hartmann's solution used to rehydrate them. This may be provided in the form of isotonic sodium bicarbonate solution (1.4% solution) or more conveniently by the use of hypertonic solutions (e.g. 8.4% solution) provided the potential dehydrating effects of using hypertonic solutions are considered and the infusion rate carefully regulated to take account of the presence of bicarbonate at the very high concentration of 1 mmol/ml. It is important when using sodium bicarbonate solutions intravenously not to mix them outside the body with calcium-containing solutions such as Hartmann's, as precipitation of calcium carbonate is likely to result. Sodium bicarbonate solutions are the treatment of choice for cases of lactic acidosis commonly seen in cattle following grain overload of the rumen. The use of lactate-containing solutions such as Hartmann's would clearly be inappropriate in these cases.

Home-prepared Hartmann's solution may be rendered more suitable for the treatment of metabolic alkalosis (e.g. in early abomasal displacement, or torsion, or vagal indigestion; Chapter 9) by the substitution of glucose for sodium lactate (Table 7.1). The addition of extra potassium ions in the form of potassium chloride is still desirable (Chapter 2), especially in long-standing cases.

References

1 Spencer, K.R. (1982) Intravenous catheters. *Veterinary Clinics of North America: Small Animal Practice* **12**, 533–43.
2 Bayly, W.M. & Vale, B.H. (1985) Intravenous catheterization and associated problems in the horse. In: *Equine Medicine and Surgery in Practice*, 26–35. Whitlock, R.H. (ed). Veterinary Learning Systems, Lawrenceville, New Jersey.
3 Corke, M.J. (1988) Economical preparation of fluids for intravenous use in cattle practice. *Veterinary Record* **122**, 305–7.
4 McDonell, W.N. (1981) General anaesthesia for gastrointestinal and obstetric procedures. *Veterinary Clinics of North America: Large Animal Practice* **3**, 163–91.

Chapter 8
Blood transfusion

Blood contains essential components for sustaining life. Transfusion is therefore indicated when lack of any or all of these components becomes a problem; they comprise erythrocytes (RBC), white blood cells (WBC), platelets and clotting factors as well as plasma.

The most common use for transfusion in veterinary practice is haemorrhagic shock, but blood may also be needed in bleeding disorders, chronic anaemias, colostrum-deprived neonates, profound hypoproteinaemia and haemolytic crises.

Matching donor with recipient requires laboratory procedures; it is important for animals requiring multiple or repeated transfusions but is seldom necessary for 'one-off' recipients. This is because unlike humans, naturally occurring isoantibody systems are relatively rare in animals. Nevertheless, records should be kept in case the need for transfusion arises again.

Blood groups

Dogs

Eight specific isoantibody systems have been identified on dog erythrocytes [1]. They are currently designated dog erythrocyte antigen (DEA) 1 to 8 (corresponding to the previously designated groups A_1, A_2, B, C, D, F, T, He) but of these only DEA 1.1 is of real clinical significance. Although all of the blood groups have the potential for stimulating the formation of specific antibodies, DEA 1.1, and to a lesser extent DEA 1.2, are the only ones to cause potentially severe reactions [2]. 63% of dogs are DEA 1.1 positive, therefore 25% of random primary transfusions could produce anti-DEA 1.1 antibodies in the recipient and so cause late haemolysis of the transfused blood and a severe immunological reaction to any subsequent transfusion. It makes sense therefore to blood type donor dogs and to avoid using DEA 1.1 or 1.2 positive blood.

Cats

The blood group system of cats is a relatively simple one. There are three specific types of blood group antigens on feline erythrocyte membranes. Two (types A and B) were originally described [3], with a new phenotype AB discovered later [4]. In Brisbane, type A has a frequency of 73.3%, B 26.3% and AB a low incidence of 0.4%.

Naturally occurring antibodies to type A occur in 95% of phenotype B cats but only 35% of type A cats have anti-B antibodies; thus there is a one-in-five possibility of a transfusion incompatibility reaction [4]. Repeated, random transfusions increase the risk of incompatibility to 37.5% and there is, clearly, a greater desirability for cross-matching before blood transfusion in cats according to these workers [4]. However, other studies [5, 6] suggest that the risk of incompatibility is not as high as the Australian workers [4] have suggested and that typing or cross-matching is probably less important than in dogs [7].

Horses

Approximately 30 factors are known in horses, segregated into eight systems (A, C, D, K, P, Q, T and U). Taken together with variation in electrophoretic forms of blood proteins, it is estimated that there are some 400 000 blood types in horses [8]. Clinically, the most important systems are A and Q, which together account for the majority of neonatal isoerythrolysis crises [10]. Both are highly antigenic and to avoid transfusion reactions and the sensitization of brood mares lacking A (usually A_1) and/or Q it is wise to select donors lacking both these factors. A is very prevalent, however, in thoroughbreds and Arabians and donors may be difficult to find in these groups. Shetlands tend to have a lower incidence of A and should be considered as donors.

Examination of the mare's serum before foaling can show whether high titres of antibodies to A_1 or Q (or less commonly R, S, E_2 and U) are present; if they are, the foal can be protected by preventing it gaining access to its mother's colostrum.

Cattle

There is a wide phenotypic variation in blood types in cattle. There are at least 11 systems with many phenogroups in each system. Cattle erythrocytes do not agglutinate well so reactions are detected by haemolysis. The J system appears to resemble the human ABO system most closely in that some cattle possess the antigen while others have only naturally occurring anti-J antibodies.

Blood groups are used extensively to establish parentage but are not of practical importance in relation to blood transfusions because single, let alone repeated transfusions are so rare. The chances of producing a sensitized animal which would be at risk to a second transfusion are therefore low.

For a fuller consideration of blood groups in cattle, sheep and pigs readers are referred to Spooner [9].

Indications for blood transfusion

Acute blood loss

A decrease in the haematocrit will decrease the oxygen-carrying capacity of the blood, though not necessarily delivery, because blood viscosity also falls.

Following haemorrhage, when replacement of circulating volume is the main requirement crystalloids or colloids can be used but, if blood loss is severe, they may cause such haemodilution that the oxygen delivery is seriously compromised. It is generally accepted that an acute fall of the PCV below 20 is an indication for a whole blood transfusion. Blood loss which occurs at the time of surgery may be estimated by swab weighing or by more sophisticated methods but if it exceeds about 18 ml/kg (roughly 20% of the estimated blood volume) it should be replaced with whole blood or red cells. Thus, not only red cells but also plasma proteins which restore oncotic pressure are provided. The volume transfused is usually around 10–20 ml/kg repeated, as required, to maintain the haematocrit above 20%. Since the transfused blood has a PCV well above 20%, additional volume replacement can still be given with crystalloids or colloids.

Anaemia

Chronic non-regenerative anaemia is a frequent indication for blood transfusion. This is not curative but merely provides the clinician with time to diagnose and attempt to treat the underlying cause. Whole blood is indicated when there are signs of anaemic anoxia which usually occur in the dog when the haematocrit falls below 15%. Cats seem able to exist at a lower haematocrit and a critical level of 12% is suggested for this species [11].

Transfusions are not used normally in the initial treatment of haemolytic anaemias but may occasionally be necessary as a life saving measure.

Bleeding disorders

Both hereditary and acquired causes of coagulopathy may be treated by the administration of whole blood, plasma or plasma components. Some factors (especially VIII and IX) and platelets are particularly labile, hence it is essential that the blood or plasma is freshly collected (a few hours old only). Thrombocytopaenias can be life-threatening and fresh blood in large volumes is needed to restore the platelet count to a reasonable level.

Severe cases of warfarin toxicity are frequently too critical to wait for a gradual build-up of vitamin K levels and these animals generally benefit from a transfusion of fresh blood or plasma; vitamin K_1 is also essential.

Hypoproteinaemia

Gross hypoproteinaemia (albumin levels below 1.5 g/dl) may require treatment with fresh plasma not only to reduce any oedema but also to reduce any bleeding tendency. Whole blood may be used as a substitute but is more likely to cause a volume overload than plasma.

Hypoproteinaemia is almost always present in severe liver disease, usually in association with a deficiency of clotting factors so that these animals have a pronounced bleeding tendency. Any surgical intervention will necessitate the administration of fresh whole blood or plasma (Chapter 12).

Choice of donors

Dogs

Blood may be obtained from live donors or collected from euthanasia cases and stored. In either case it must be collected aseptically.

Live donors should be of a reasonable size (at least 25–30 kg) and physically fit. Greyhounds because of their temperament and morphology make ideal donors. Either sex may be used, although if females are chosen, they should be spayed, in order to negate the influence of oestrogens on platelets. The animals should have a haematocrit of at least 40% and ideally should be DEA 1.1 and DEA 1.2 negative (A −ve in old classification).

Depending on the requirements of the clinic and the number of donors kept, animals may either be bled as needed or bled regularly and the blood stored for future use. The advantage of the former system is that the blood is always fresh but this system requires more dogs to be kept for a given volume requirement of blood.

In the absence of live donors, practices may wish to collect blood from anaesthetized dogs before euthanasia (with the owner's full consent). Although this allows large volumes of blood to be collected from each dog, the disadvantages are that the animal may not be healthy, the blood will inevitably contain drugs and this blood may become outdated more rapidly. It is certainly not likely to be of use in situations where clotting factors are required.

Cats

Donor cats should be mature and large but not obese. There is no breed preference but a docile nature is helpful. Blood typing is not generally performed because of the lack of commercially available antisera but the haematocrit should be checked and ideally should be at least 35%.

It is important that both dogs and cats kept as donors are provided with a diet adequate in vitamins, minerals and proteins. Dietary supplementation with iron, B_{12}, folic acid, pyridoxine has been suggested by some workers [12].

Practical aspects of collection

The easiest and safest site for venepuncture in live donors (both dogs and cats) is the jugular vein. In cases destined for euthanasia, the femoral or carotid artery may be cannulated for rapid exsanguination. Repeated cannulation of arteries produces scarring and is not recommended for live donors. Local anaesthetic should be infiltrated at the site of venepuncture in conscious donors and large-bore needles should be used. The site should always be thoroughly cleansed as for surgery. An alternative method of collection is cardiac puncture. It is, however, potentially very dangerous and is not advised unless the animal is destined for euthanasia.

The blood should be collected into a container with the appropriate amount of anticoagulant and this should be rotated gently during collection so that blood and anticoagulant are mixed. If a vacuum system is used to speed collection in large animals, it is very important that the blood is not allowed to 'jet' on to the bottom of the container, otherwise the red cells will be damaged. Nowadays, proprietary blood collecting kits are easily the most convenient means of collecting blood from dogs (Fig. 8.1). They contain sufficient coagulant, usually CPD (citrate phosphate dextrose) for 500 ml of blood and have integral collection tubing and needle (Fenwal Laboratories).

Unsedated, healthy live donors can safely be used to give 10–20 ml/kg blood every 10 days or so [13], although in an emergency, provided the volume collected is replenished with some form of plasma substitute, greater quantities may be collected.

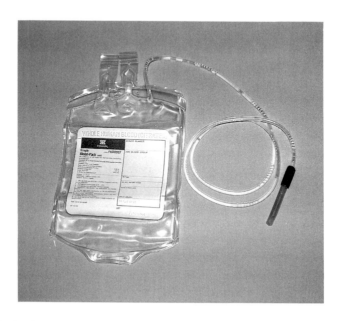

Fig. 8.1 Blood collection bag.

Storage

Various anticoagulants are available to prevent coagulation — acid citrate dextrose (ACD), citrate phosphate dextrose (CPD), ethylenediaminetetra-acetic acid (EDTA) and heparin, but if heparin or EDTA is used, the blood must be used immediately. Heparin (20–30 mg/500 ml) may be useful when collecting small volumes for immediate infusion into very small dogs or cats. Citrated blood should not be mixed with 'Haemaccel' or other calcium-containing solutions though they can be used consecutively but only if the infusion line is flushed with saline in between.

CPD is preferred to ACD because red cell viability is prolonged to 4 weeks compared to 3 weeks in ACD [14]; moreover large amounts of ACD may cause metabolic acidosis. Cats, however, are sensitive to citrate and the final concentration should not exceed 0.4% [15]. Blood should always be stored at 4°C as storage at higher temperatures dramatically reduces post-infusion red cell viability [16].

Storage lesions

Storage of blood results in several biochemical changes which reduce the quality of the blood. The main limit on storage time is post-transfusion red cell viability; it is generally believed that at least 70% of transfused cells should still be viable 24 hours later to be useful.

Red cell viability is closely related to ATP levels in human blood although canine cells may be less dependent on ATP [14]. Levels of 2,3-diphosphoglycerate (2,3-DPG) also drop during storage, thus with time the haemoglobin–oxygen dissociation curve moves to the left, i.e. oxygen affinity increases and oxygen release to tissues becomes more difficult; in severely ill animals this could be critical.

Blood pH also decreases during storage and this also shifts the haemoglobin dissociation curve (to the right); however the effect on the recipient is usually minimal. Other storage changes include a fall in P_{O_2}, glucose and bicarbonate levels and a rise in P_{CO_2} and lactate. Intra and extracellular potassium and sodium also tend to equilibrate so that plasma $[K^+]$ tends to rise but this change is minimal in dog blood compared to human blood [17], because canine RBC are low in K^+ (like those of cats, most cattle and sheep, but not horses).

Red cells become rigid and fragile during storage and haemolysis is much more likely. White cells, platelets and clotting factors rarely survive more than 24 hours and micro-aggregates of these constituents begin to develop very quickly. The number of micro-aggregates increases dramatically after the first week of storage and by the end of the third week there may be 100×10^6 micro-aggregates ranging in size from $10-40\,\mu m$ in each unit of blood. Infusion of large numbers of these aggregates predisposes to pulmonary capillary damage and pulmonary oedema and old, stored blood should always be filtered through a $20\,\mu m$ diameter filter before administration.

Cross-matching blood

Cross-matching will detect incompatibility between donor and recipient and is essential if the recipient is suspected of being previously sensitized. Two types of match should be carried out, major and minor. The major test determines the compatibility of donor cells with recipient serum, i.e. does the recipient have antibodies to the donor cells? The minor match tests the compatibility of donor serum and recipient cells, i.e. does the donor have antibodies to recipient cells? Both tests must be performed on fresh blood. Exact details vary from laboratory to laboratory but the broad technique is the same. Five millilitres of blood are collected from both donor and recipient and allowed to clot. A red cell suspension (5%) of each clot is prepared in saline (0.5 ml cells + 9.5 ml saline) and the following tests are carried out in separate test tubes:

1 0.1 ml of donor cell suspension + 0.1 ml recipient serum (major).
2 0.1 ml of recipient cell suspension + 0.1 ml donor serum (minor).
3 0.1 ml of donor cell suspension + 0.1 ml donor serum (control).
4 0.1 ml of recipient cell suspension + 0.1 ml recipient serum (control).

Each test is done in duplicate or triplicate and incubated for up to an hour at 37°C. One set is often also incubated at 4°C to check for cold agglutination.

After incubation the tubes are gently centrifuged and the supernatants checked for haemolysis. The cells are then checked for signs of agglutination. Gross agglutination will be evident as a clot but minor clumping will only be detected by resuspending the cells and examining on a *warm* slide under a microscope.

Any degree of major match incompatibility is a contraindication to carrying out the transfusion; a minor cross-match reaction is more difficult to evaluate and may be tolerated in an emergency.

Administration of blood

Blood that has been stored in a refrigerator should be warmed *slowly* to room temperature before administration. The bags should be inverted gently several times to resuspend the red cells but should not be shaken violently. Active heating of the bag of blood should be avoided because temperatures above 45°C induce clotting, but if the blood is required quickly it may be warmed as it passes through the coiled tubing of the giving set (Fig. 8.2) by immersing this in a warm (38−40°C) water bath. Cold blood should not be infused; it is more viscous and therefore takes longer to transfuse, it provokes vasoconstriction, lowers body temperature and may also produce cardiac arrhythmias.

Sterile disposable giving sets suitable for blood administration are readily available. All incorporate large nylon net filters of 170−200 μm pore size, suitable for filtering large clots and particles and some include a device for infusion under manual pressure. These standard sets will not remove micro-aggregates, however, and for this purpose special micropore filters (pore size 20 μm) will be required (Plate 4).

To reduce the viscosity of the blood and hence facilitate its infusion in young puppies and kittens it may mixed with normal saline so that it flows more freely through fine (23 G) catheters. Blood should not be mixed with Ca^{++}-containing solutions (e.g. Hartmann's) if a calcium-binding anticoagulant (e.g. citrate) has been used.

Blood is usually given via the jugular or cephalic veins but in

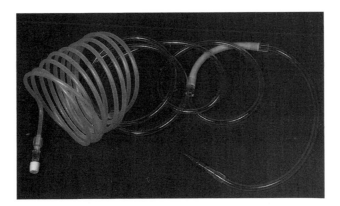

Fig. 8.2 Infusion coil for warming i.v. solution.

neonates intraperitoneal infusion may be the only route possible; however, absorption of blood by this route is extremely slow (40% in 24 hours) and it cannot be recommended except in a dire emergency. The presence of peritonitis will preclude the use of this route. The intramedullary infusion of blood is often mentioned as a possible alternative to intravenous infusion but it has never been used by the authors and it is hard to imagine that this route is a practical proposition.

Initially, the infusion should be slow and the patient watched carefully for any signs of transfusion reactions. If after 20−30 minutes there are no problems the rate of infusion may then be increased. A useful formula relating the desired PCV to the volume of blood required [18] is:

$$V = \left[W \times \frac{D - P}{T} \right] \times 90 \text{ (dog) } or \times 70 \text{ (cat)}$$

where V = ml of blood needed, W = patient's weight (kg), D = desired PCV, P = patient's PCV, and T = transfusion PCV.

Once a pack of blood has been opened or warmed it should be used within 24 hours to reduce the possibility of bacterial contamination.

Hazards of transfusion

Incompatibility

Transfusion reactions can vary in severity from life-threatening hae-molytic crises to mild urticaria which may respond to intramuscular antihistamine injections or not need treatment at all. They may be immunologically or non-immunologically mediated.

Severe reactions produce immediate hypotension, vomiting, fever, salivation, haemolysis and haemoglobinuria and consumption of clotting factors can lead to coagulopathy. Milder reactions result in delayed, slight jaundice and anaemia. In the most severe form, death occurs some 1−3 days later as a result of acute renal failure due to renal tubular damage, but this is not invariable and dogs often make good recoveries after quite severe haemolytic reactions.

Cats rarely show transfusion reactions partly because they are often immunosuppressed by the disease for which they are being treated — e.g. FeLV infection.

Pyrogenic reactions

Fever may be produced by the presence of recipient antibodies to donor white cells or platelets or because of the presence of pyrogens in the equipment. Reactions to pyrogens often develop within 20–30 minutes. *Bacterial contamination* may also cause a fever. Warming blood will allow any bacteria present to multiply and septicaemia can develop very quickly. Thrombophlebitis at the catheter site can also precipitate septicaemia, however, and this should always be checked.

Circulatory overload

This may be a problem in those patients with cardiac or renal problems and dogs in heart failure are unable to tolerate infusions greater than 4 ml/kg/hour. Chronically anaemic animals are also at risk. If the heart is unable to cope, CVP rises and pulmonary congestion develops. Clinically these animals become dyspnoeic, cyanosed, start coughing and may also start vomiting and develop urticaria. It is essential to transfuse susceptible animals slowly and to treat promptly should any signs develop. Measures include diuresis and vasodilation together with the possible use of suitable inotropic agents.

Biochemical effects

Reduction in ionized calcium

The rapid transfusion of large volumes of stored blood may cause citrate intoxication. Normally, the liver is able to metabolize citrate rapidly but if there is liver damage or the infusion is very fast hepatic metabolism may be unable to keep pace. The citrate will then chelate calcium and allow signs of hypocalcaemia to develop (muscle tetany/tremors, cardiac arrhythmias). In extreme cases, i.e. massive transfusion, there will also be interference with clotting. Treatment involves the slow intravenous administration of calcium gluconate (10 ml of 10% solution/l of transfused blood) or calcium chloride (6 ml of 10% $CaCl_2$/500 ml transfused blood).

Acidosis

It was formerly thought that since stored blood becomes acid due to high lactic acid and carbon dioxide contents, massive transfusion would give rise to an acidosis in the recipient. However, the carbon dioxide is excreted in the first passage through the lungs and the lactate is rapidly metabolized in the liver. This metabolism of lactate together with that of the citrate anticoagulant produces bicarbonate which, until it is excreted in the kidneys, results in alkalosis. Thus, alkalosis is the normal result of the massive transfusion of stored blood and acidosis is only seen if transfusion is inadequate and results in impaired tissue perfusion and hypoxic lactic acidosis.

Reduction of 2,3-DPG levels

2,3-diphosphoglycerate (2,3-DPG) is an intermediary in the glycolytic pathway and its deficiency shifts the oxygen dissociation curve to the left, so reducing oxygen release to the tissues. ACD anticoagulant causes the 2,3-DPG levels to fall to about half of normal in about 5 days, to less than 25% after 10 days and to less than 10% after 3 weeks. Loss of 2,3-DPG is only half as fast when CPD anticoagulant is used and the addition of adenine reduces the loss still further so that commercially available packs for blood collection and storage now generally contain a CPD−adenine anticoagulant mixture.

Coagulation defects (see reduction in ionized calcium, p. 159)

Stored blood is platelet deficient but thrombocytopenia from massive blood transfusion is seldom a cause of coagulation defects. However, massive transfusions of stored blood could, theoretically, cause a bleeding problem either via hypocalcaemia or by diluting factors V and VIII. This may become a problem when the rate of transfusion is greater than 1 ml/kg/minute (as it may have to be in treating massive sudden haemorrhage). Failure of haemostasis is not seen until levels of factors V and VIII are less than about 30% of normal and the fresher the transfused blood the less likely will a coagulation defect due to this cause be encountered since even after 21 days of storage blood may contain 20−50% of the normal levels of these factors.

In cases where factors V and VIII are reduced below the haemostatic level there will be an increase in prothrombin time and partial thromboplastin time or kaolin cephalin coagulation time. Treatment is by infusion of *fresh* plasma/blood.

Disease transmission

This is a possibility but may be minimized by keeping donors and monitoring them regularly for any potentially transmissible disease.

Air embolism

This is only a danger when rigid bottles are used for the blood. Thus, it is now rarely a danger.

Autologous blood transfusion

Reinfusion of the animal's own blood may be a safe, cost effective and preferable alternative to homologous transfusions in many veterinary situations. The technique is not new, having been used in man as long ago as 1874 [19], but it has only recently been 'rediscovered' by medical workers. Autologous blood eliminates the danger of transfusion reactions and disease transmission. There are three techniques of autologous blood transfusion:

1 Pre-operative collection and storing.
2 Acute peri-operative collection and haemodilution.
3 Intra-operative blood scavenging and recycling.

In elective surgery where large blood losses are anticipated, blood may be collected 1−2 weeks pre-operatively and stored at 4°C in CPD or ACD. In patients with good bone marrow responses and adequate vitamin B_{12} and iron supplementation, these RBC are replaced in 7−10 days and the haematocrit should be back to normal. The stored blood can then be used during surgery when losses begin.

Alternatively, blood may be collected, acutely, immediately before surgery, after the induction of anaesthesia. The volume taken is made up by equal amounts of a synthetic colloid solution (Haemaccel or dextran 70) so that normovolaemic haemodilution is achieved. The haematocrit is lowered to 30−35% thus improving microcirculatory flow by reducing the viscosity of the blood. As the patient bleeds intra-operatively, further blood which is lost will be 'dilute' and is then replaced by the autologous units which are reinfused in reverse order of collection from the most dilute to the most concentrated.

The third technique involves the collection and recycling of shed blood during surgery. The main obstacle to this method is the problem of collecting, anticoagulating and cleansing the shed blood efficiently and easily. Systems are available for humans but they are expensive and unlikely to be practicable in veterinary practice. Alternatively, blood can be collected from opened body cavities by sterile syringe or by gentle suction and quickly transferred into bags containing anticoagulant. Blood collected in this way should always be infused via a filter to remove any particulate matter. In an emergency, blood can even be salvaged from saturated swabs by washing them in sterile saline and then centrifuging the liquid (or letting it settle). The supernatant is discarded and the cells can then be reconstituted in Hartmann's and reinfused via a micropore filter.

Excessive haemolysis due to mechanical damage of the red cells may occur if excessive suction or agitation is used in collecting shed blood. When this occurs the blood should not be used as renal failure is likely to occur. Thrombocytopenia is also a potential problem and ideally some homologous blood should be available to counteract this.

A variation on the collection of shed blood involves the collection of blood from a closed body cavity following an episode of bleeding due to trauma. The blood can be collected by aspiration into syringes or into blood collection bags and then reinfused via a micropore filter (20 μm). No anticoagulant is needed if the blood has been in contact with serous surfaces for 45 minutes or more as the mechanical movement of the heart and lungs and contact with peritoneal surfaces causes defibrination and platelet destruction [20]. If the haemorrhage has just occurred CPD (37 ml/500 ml blood) or heparin should be used to prevent coagulation.

Autotransfusion is not safe if the blood is contaminated with urine, faeces, fat, bile, pus or neoplastic cells and blood which has been present in the body cavity for over 24 hours. Old shed blood contains too many micro-aggregates and will be too haemolysed for safe use. Reinfusion of blood containing large numbers of micro-aggregates is likely to provoke disseminated intravascular coagulation (DIC) and also pulmonary capillary damage leading to pulmonary oedema, 'shock lung' [21]. Micropore filters will remove microemboli but not the vasoactive amines liberated by platelet aggregation and it is these substances which contribute to the development of 'shock lung' as well as producing bronchoconstriction. Thrombocytopenia is also a problem in recycled blood as platelet aggregation is precipitated by contact with serous surfaces and air.

There are obvious hazards associated with scavenging of shed blood but when large volumes have been lost and haemorrhage persists it is often the only way that the requirement for blood can be met.

Use of blood products

Separating blood into its various components is widely practised in human medicine because it makes the most efficient use of the blood. In the veterinary field it is not widely used mainly because of the need for access to blood bank centrifuges.

Plasma

Plasma may be decanted from sedimented blood (allow to settle over a few hours) and stored in sterile containers. It may be stored for up to a year at very low temperatures or about 3 months in a household freezer compartment.

Plasma is indicated in animals with hypoproteinaemia or hypovolaemia not caused by acute blood loss. It is also a useful source of antibodies for neonates with failure of passive transfer from the dam and, for example, in foals, 1 litre is likely to provide immunoglobulin G (IgG) levels in plasma above 400 mg/dl [22]. Fresh plasma is also a source of coagulation factors which may be used to treat DIC but must be harvested and frozen within a few hours of collection, if it is to be useful for this purpose.

Packed red cells

In the UK, plasma and anticoagulant are removed from collected blood by centrifuging blood gently or by allowing the cells to settle over several hours. This leaves a suspension having a haematocrit of about 70% which is called 'plasma-reduced blood'. In the USA this preparation is usually referred to as 'packed red cells' — a term reserved in the UK for a more concentrated suspension with a haematocrit of 70−80% which is seldom used today. The use of plasma-reduced blood (whatever it is called) has much to commend it. It contains as many erythrocytes as whole blood and is, therefore, equally useful for improving blood oxygen transport while, at the same time, supplies of plasma are made available for use in other cases. There is, however, no point in transfusing blood or plasma-reduced blood to increase plasma volume; it is time-consuming (i.e. expensive) to produce and crystalloid solutions, albumin solutions or plasma substitutes are equally effective. Plasma-reduced blood can be 'reconstituted' by adding 200 ml of normal saline to each 300 ml using a Y-infusion set. This is routine practice in centres where the reduction in viscosity achieved by dilution is considered to be advantageous in improving the flow rate possible through an infusion apparatus. However, even without dilution, flow rates are usually acceptably rapid through any cannula larger than size 16 FG. Packed cells are used to transfuse animals with anaemia in which whole blood would cause dangerous circulatory overload.

Cryoprecipitate plasma

This is obtained by thawing fresh frozen plasma at 4°C and separating out the resulting cold precipitated material. This material is rich in the antihaemophilic factor, Von Willebrand's factor and fibrinogen and if deep frozen, can be kept for about a year.

Platelets

Low speed centrifugation of fresh blood (375 × g for 15 minutes) produces plasma rich in platelets and is indicated in cases of severe thrombocytopaenia as well as DIC.

Artificial blood

Blood is no longer the safe, readily available fluid it once was in human medicine. This has intensified the pressures to develop totally artificial blood substitutes. The early ones have used fluorocarbons as oxygen carriers [23] but suffer from the drawback of needing an oxygen enriched atmosphere. Clearly, it will not be long before satisfactory substitutes are developed and eventually, once price and availability allow, they are likely to find extensive applications in veterinary medicine as there should be no species specificity involved in their use.

References

1 Pichler, M. & Turnwald, G.H. (1985) Blood transfusion in the dog and cat. Part I. Physiology, collection, storage and indication for whole blood therapy. *Compendium of Continuing Education for the Practising Veterinarian* **7**, 64−71.

2 Moore, D.J. (1976) The blood grouping system of dogs. *Journal of the South African Veterinary Association* **47**, 282—3.

3 Eyquem, A.L. Podliachouk, L. & Milot, P. (1962) Blood groups in chimpanzees, horses, sheep and pigs and other mammals. *Annals of the New York Academy of Science* **97**, 320—8.

4 Auer, L. & Bell, K. (1981) The AB blood group system of cats. *Animal Blood Groups and Biochemical Genetics* **12**(4), 287—97.

5 Hayes, A., Mastrota, F., Mooney, S. & Hurvitz, A. (1982) Safety of transfusing blood in cats. *Journal of the American Veterinary Medical Association* **181**, 4—5.

6 Cotter, S.M. (1982) Blood transfusion reactions in cats. *Journal of the American Veterinary Medical Association* **181**, 5—6.

7 Kitchell, B.E. & Haskins, S.C. (1984) Feline trauma and critical care medicine. *Veterinary Clinics of North America: Small Animal Practice* **14**, 1331—44.

8 Stormont, C. (1979) Positive horse identification. Part II Blood typing. *Equine Practice* **1**, 48—54.

9 Spooner, R.L. (1980) Blood groups in animals. In: *Scientific Foundations of Veterinary Medicine*, 421—7. Phillipson, A.T., Hall, L.W. & Pritchard, W.R. (eds). Heinemann, London.

10 Stormont, C. (1975) Neonatal isoerythrolysis in domestic animals: A comparative review. In: *Advances in Veterinary Science and Comparative Medicine*, 23—43. Brandley, C.A. & Cornelius, C.E. (eds). Academic Press, New York. Vol. **19**.

11 Penman, V. & Schall, W.D. (1983) Diseases of the red blood cells. In: *Textbook of Veterinary Medicine*, 1938—2000. Ettinger, S.J. (ed). W.B. Saunders, Philadelphia.

12 Greene, C.E. (1982) Blood transfusion therapy: an updated overview. *Proceedings of the 49th Annual Meeting of the American Animal Hospital Association* South Bend, Indiana 187—9.

13 Potkay, S. & Zinn, R.D. (1969) Effect of collection material, bodyweight and season on the hemograms of canine blood donors. *Laboratory Animal Care* **19**, 192.

14 Eisenbrandt, D.L. & Smith, J.E. (1973) Evaluation of preservatives and containers for storage of canine blood. *Journal of the American Veterinary Medical Association* **163**, 988—90.

15 Clark, C.H. (1983) In: *Feline Medicine*, 51—3. Pratt, P.W. (ed). American Veterinary Publications Inc., Santa Barbara.

16 Shields, C.E. (1972) Application of isotopic methods for measuring post transfusion survival of stored blood in dogs. *Laboratory Animal Science* **22**, 196—202.

17 Owen, R.ap R. & Holmes, P.H. (1972) An assessment of the viability of canine blood stored under normal veterinary hospital conditions. *Veterinary Record* **90**, 231—6.

18 Killingworth, C.R. (1984) Use of blood and blood components for feline and canine patients. *Journal of the American Veterinary Medical Association* **185**, 1452—5.

19 Isbister, J.P. & Davis, R. (1980) Should autologous blood transfusion be rediscovered? *Anaesthesia and Intensive Care Journal* **8** Part II, 168—71.

20 Turnwald, G.H. & Pichler, M.E. (1985) Blood transfusion in dogs and cats. Part II. Administration, adverse effects, and component therapy. *Compendium of Continuing Education for the Practising Veterinarian* **7**, 115—24.

21 Crowe, D.T. (1980) Autotransfusion in the trauma patient. *Veterinary Clinics of North America: Small Animal Practice* Symposium on Trauma **10** Part III, 581—97.

22 Becht, J.L. & Gordon, B.J. (1987) Blood and plasma therapy. In: *Current Therapy in Equine Medicine* Part II, 317—22. W.B. Saunders, Philadelphia.

23 Wickham, N.W.R. & Hardy, R.N. (1982) Artificial blood from flourocarbons. *Hospital Update* **8**, 1433—44.

Chapter 9
Fluid therapy for gastrointestinal disturbances

Introduction

The intestinal tract, as the site for normal water, electrolyte and nutrient absorption, is where disease can cause profound disturbances to the normal state of hydration and electrolyte balance. Disturbance can result from diarrhoea, vomiting, intestinal malabsorption, or obstruction, and the consequences in terms of abnormal function can occur rapidly and require early treatment. For most gastrointestinal disturbances, fluid therapy is either desirable or essential as part of the treatment regime. Indeed, gastrointestinal disorders probably provide the most frequent indication for veterinary fluid therapy.

Normal fluid exchange in the gastrointestinal tract

In a healthy animal, fluid is taken in by mouth, either as liquid or as water included in food. From this point onwards, a series of water movements occurs in and out of the lumen, either resulting in a net addition (e.g. in the stomach), or in a net absorption (e.g. in the small intestine or colon). Figure 9.1 summarizes the movements diagrammatically. In the healthy animal, overall intake by the mouth is balanced by losses through faeces, skin, lungs, and most important, kidney.

Within the animal, net endogenous secretion of saliva, gastric juice, pancreatic juice, and bile is balanced by net absorption lower down the small intestine or the colon. The situation is further complicated by bi-directional fluxes which occur at all points in the intestine. These can be measured using isotopes, and are large in comparison with net movements. Thus, the water flux towards and from the intestine in a healthy calf can be estimated at about 90–100 l/day, while the net absorption is only about 3–4 l [1]. As a result of the magnitude of these fluxes, small changes in their balance can cause major disruption and a change from normal net uptake of

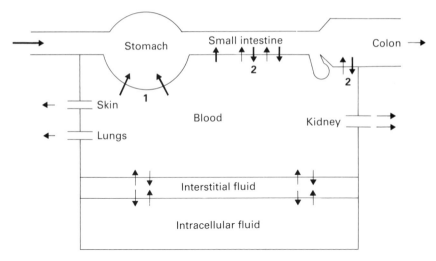

Fig. 9.1 Normal fluid balance: (1) net secretion; (2) net absorption.

water to abnormal net secretion of water and resulting dehydration. The converse is, however, that an increase in net uptake (such as that resulting from oral rehydration) can be used to treat dehydration.

The role played by the colon is of particular interest. The kidney has long been recognized as an organ of compensation which is concerned with regulation of water and electrolyte balance. The colon should also be considered in the same role, and even responds to the same mediator, namely aldosterone, by conserving water and sodium at the expense of potassium [2]. In the normal animal, the colon regulates the consistency of the material leaving it (faeces), and can compensate for some degree of small intestinal malfunction or hypersecretion. Where diarrhoea occurs, the colonic compensation has been overcome. Alternatively, the colon itself may be the origin of diarrhoea, as occurs in swine dysentery [3].

Vomiting

Vomiting may be caused by localized gastritis, alimentary obstruction or it may be a symptom of a general toxaemia such as that associated with pyometra or kidney disease [4]. Where gastritis and inflammation are present this may change the constituents of the secretion, with proportionally larger losses of serum, protein, and possibly whole blood.

There are distinct variations between species in their ability to vomit, and in the ease with which vomiting can occur. Rodents and horses do not vomit, while dogs and cats vomit with an ease which verges on the casual. The latter species use the reflex as a protection against accidental ingestion of irritant material. Vomiting carries the risk of excessive fluid and electrolyte loss where it is prolonged by gastritis, so producing continual stimulation of the reflex.

Mechanism of vomiting

Irritation of gastric mucosa leads to stimulation of afferent fibres leading to the vomiting centre situated in the medulla. This is also influenced by impulses from the chemoreceptor trigger zone (CTZ) on the floor of the third ventricle. The CTZ can be stimulated by circulatory toxins, as in pyometra, or by uraemia following kidney failure. In the latter case, a contributory factor may be failure to eliminate circulating gastrin, which produces hypersecretion of acid via H_2 receptor stimulation. This may lead to mucosal irritation and further stimulation of vomiting.

Metabolic consequence of vomiting (Figure 9.2)

Continual vomiting causes losses of H^+ and Cl^-, and so eventually a metabolic alkalosis may be predicted. However, more commonly in mild to moderate vomiting, a metabolic *acidosis* is encountered [5]. The reasons for this apparent paradox may include: loss of alkaline duodenal content, loss of bicarbonate in simultaneous diarrhoea, or compensation by the kidney for H^+ loss in vomit. Metabolic alkalosis *is* seen where there is pyloric obstruction, or where vomiting is profuse and frequent. The acid loss then results in abnormally high plasma bicarbonate with a rise in plasma pH. The low chloride concentration leads to bicarbonate conservation with sodium in the kidney, which aggravates the alkalosis. Meanwhile, potassium excretion is increased by aldosterone in exchange for conserved sodium (Chapter 2).

Fluid therapy in vomiting

An attempt should be made to estimate the continuing fluid losses which are occurring and to replace the existing deficit by the parenteral

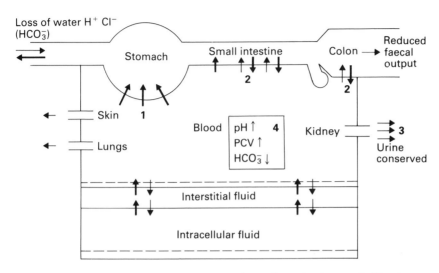

Fig. 9.2 Severe vomiting: (1) secretion increased; (2) absorption increased; (3) urine conserved; (4) alkalosis (severe vomiting). Acidosis is often seen in mild cases.

route [5]. It is often the case that the amount of fluid lost will be underestimated, and so the volume given should be suitably increased to allow for this.

The subcutaneous route is suitable only when a mild deficit is present, while the oral route using an appropriate rehydration fluid may be suitable despite the vomiting. This is because sufficient of the ingested fluid will usually be retained to give benefit to the patient, especially if the fluid is offered in relatively small quantities [6]. Vomiting in itself, therefore, is *not* a contraindication for oral fluid replacement (though its cause may be), but progress must be carefully monitored to ensure that parenteral treatment can indeed be avoided.

Parenteral rehydration is the route of choice where facilities allow. The choice of rehydration solution ideally depends on knowledge of the physiological state of the animal. As stated above, acidosis is often encountered and a solution such as Hartmann's is generally suitable unless the acidosis is severe.

In severe vomiting (e.g. pyloric stenosis) which can result in metabolic alkalosis, one should avoid the toxic acidifying salts such as NH_4Cl, since the condition can be satisfactorily treated by rehydrating the animal with Ringer's solution or 0.9% saline, which will be followed by renal correction of the alkalosis (Chapter 2). Such animals may require additional potassium (20 mmol/l) in the rehydration fluid.

Diarrhoea

Diarrhoea threatens any child or young animal existing in conditions of poor hygiene. This inevitably includes many situations on farms and in kennels, where exposure of individuals to faecal material from other animals cannot be avoided. When diarrhoea occurs in young animals, the resulting drain on fluid and electrolyte reserves is particularly likely to be life-threatening. By contrast, adult animals can withstand the losses unless exceptionally severe, e.g. those associated with parvovirus infection in dogs and cats, or cholera in man.

The loss of water and electrolyte in the small intestine can be partially offset by increased absorption in the large intestine [1]. Absorption in the colon is stimulated by aldosterone, secreted in response to volume depletion [7].

Enterotoxic (secretory) diarrhoea

Diarrhoea can result from a number of bacterial infections, the best known being enterotoxigenic *Escherichia coli* (ETEC), and *Salmonella*. Numerous other bacteria have, however, been associated with diarrhoea, although their exact role is unclear.

E. coli was for many years linked with diarrhoea in young animals, but the pathogenesis remained questionable until it was demonstrated that certain strains of the organism produced enterotoxins which were capable of stimulating the intestinal mucosa to secrete water and electrolyte [8]. This was shown to occur with little change in mucosal structure, and since their identification, a considerable amount of information is now available concerning the nature, the structure, and the mode of action of the toxins produced by *E. coli*. The main division between the toxins is between heat labile toxin (LT) and heat stable toxin (ST). LT has a high molecular weight, is strongly antigenic, and in many ways resembles the cholera toxin. ST has a low molecular weight and can be further subdivided into ST_A and ST_B, the former being more active in neonatal piglets, the latter being more active in weaned piglets [9].

The mode of action of the two toxins at the cellular level has been distinguished in that heat stable toxin has been shown to affect formation of cyclic guanosine monophosphate (GMP) [10], while the heat stable toxin, like cholera toxin, affects cyclic adenosine mono-phosphate (AMP) [11]. This is shown diagrammatically in Fig. 9.3. This also shows that the final secretion is further influenced by cal-modulin (calcium dependent regulator) and that the net result is a secretion of chloride and sodium ions, with accompanying water.

The fluid secreted into the intestine following enterotoxin stimu-lation closely resembles ECF, and the main losses are of sodium, chloride, bicarbonate, potassium and water. The main site of losses is in the distal small intestine where the ETEC attach and colonize in large numbers owing to their possession of attachment antigens such as the K88 and 987P (common among pig ETEC), and K99 (common among calf ETEC). The resulting fluid movements are shown in Fig. 9.4. The losses in the small intestine may partly be compensated in the large intestine, but where diarrhoea results, this compensatory capacity is overwhelmed.

Salmonellosis may also involve hypersecretion because some strains do produce enterotoxins [12]; however local inflammation within the intestinal mucosa is an additional factor. This may itself be sufficient to account for the fluid loss through secretory prostaglandins.

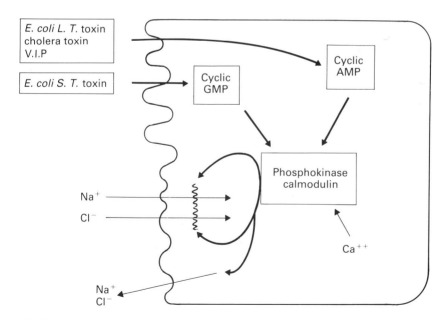

Fig. 9.3 Diarrhoeic secretion.

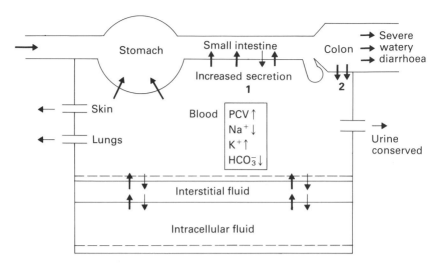

Fig. 9.4 Diarrhoea — enterotoxic: (1) increased secretion; (2) increased absorption.

Malabsorptive diarrhoea

This is typically caused by rotavirus, coronavirus, cryptosporidia and parvovirus. In most species, rotavirus is almost as ubiquitous as *E. coli* and can cause loss of the upper section of the villus, with consequent depression in brush-border enzymes, particularly disaccharidases such as lactase [13]. This is particularly important in the young animal where lactose is the main source of carbohydrate. Lactose can be absorbed only after hydrolysis to glucose and galactose, which are actively absorbed by the intestinal mucosa. Coronavirus and crypto-sporidia appear to be responsible for greater destruction of villous structure than rotavirus, while parvovirus infection in dogs (and pan-leucopenia infection in cats) can cause a complete loss of the mucosa, including crypts [14]. Rotavirus affects the small intestinal mucosa, but coronavirus can damage the mucosa of both small and large intestine [15].

Malabsorptive (e.g. viral) diarrhoea results from several factors (Fig. 9.5). Firstly, the area available for absorption of nutrients will be reduced by the loss of villi. Secondly, the remaining crypt cells tend to be net secretors rather than net absorbers. Thirdly, the loss of the villus tips, even in mild malabsorptive diarrhoea, results in loss of those mature enterocytes most able to digest disaccharides.

Undigested carbohydrate reaching the colon will be fermented by

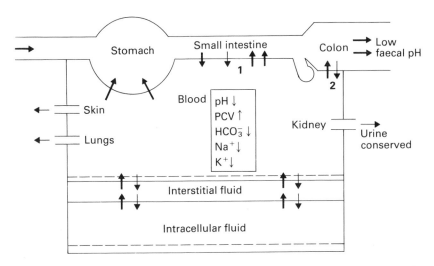

Fig. 9.5 Diarrhoea — malabsorptive rotavirus infection: (1) malabsorption; (2) osmotic secretion following fermentation.

the resident flora to small, osmotically active, particles such as short chain fatty acids [13]. Water is therefore drawn into the lumen, and diarrhoea results. However, there is clearly some reserve capacity of disaccharidase activity, and lactose intolerance is not always seen in rotavirus infection [16]. Furthermore, fermentation of carbohydrate to fatty acid is a normal feature of colon function in pigs and horses, so that, at least in these species, further factors may operate. Among these are the toxic amines, e.g. putrescine and cadaverine, which may result from protein breakdown by colonic bacteria [17].

Interaction between virus and ETEC

In calves and pigs, the relative importance of secretory and malabsorptive diarrhoea remains a matter of debate. Surveys suggest that in calves uncomplicated ETEC diarrhoea is seldom found in animals greater than 3 days of age [18]. In older animals, rotavirus, coronavirus, or cryptosporidia are more frequently identified as the primary cause; however rotavirus (by far the most common of the three) causes relatively mild diarrhoea, and severe disease only occurs when it combines with ETEC [19].

Dehydration

Disturbances of body fluids are dealt with in Chapter 2 and their clinical and laboratory manifestations in Chapter 5. The visible changes are of major importance to the clinician. The classic symptoms of dehydration (sunken eye, tight skin, etc.) are seen only when the animal has lost about 5% of its body weight, i.e. is already significantly dehydrated. It is therefore important to treat animals, not merely according to gross symptoms, but to take into account the likely deficit even when overt symptoms are mild or absent.

Routes of rehydration in diarrhoea

Oral rehydration

This technique allows restoration of circulatory volume and correction of deficits without recourse to parenteral routes of administration. The basis of the technique is shown diagrammatically in Fig. 9.6.

Glucose and neutral amino acids are absorbed actively in separate mechanisms by the mucosal cells in the small intestine. The absorption of both glucose [20] and amino acid [21] is sodium-dependent, and thus linked absorption occurs from the lumen to the cell. Sodium is then actively extruded into the intercellular space, and the glucose or amino acid also passes out of the cell. The resulting raised osmolality within the interstitial fluid causes water movement through the intercellular junction (the 'tight' junction) [22]. Finally, the water, together with the electrolytes, glucose and amino acid, enters the circulation. Thus, glucose and some amino acids, at suitable concentrations, can promote sodium and water uptake from the gut, even during diarrhoea; the anions of certain fatty acids have similar effects.

The above mechanism is not affected by enterotoxins from *E. coli*, despite the secretion caused by such toxins [23]. Viral or malabsorptive diarrhoea leaves intact sufficient absorptive capacity to benefit from oral rehydration [24]. Indeed, in humans, even some parasitic diarrhoeas may benefit [25].

The importance of oral rehydration was first recognized in the treatment of cholera victims [26], where it has been dramatically effective in reducing mortality and has almost totally superseded intravenous therapy. An effective oral rehydration solution (ORS) should contain the ingredients shown in Fig. 9.7.

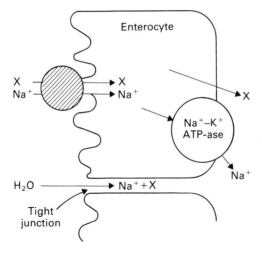

Fig. 9.6 Oral rehydration: x = glucose or amino acid.

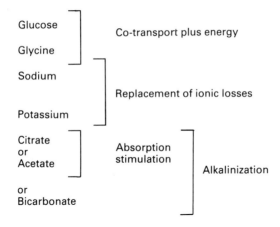

Fig. 9.7 Typical formulation for oral rehydration.

The osmolality of available oral rehydration solutions is usually approximately isotonic (300 mOsm/kg). However, it has been suggested that hypertonic solutions may be used [27] where increased amounts of glucose are added in order to make the energy content more comparable with milk. Such solutions may cause an initial fluid secretion to produce lumen isotonicity before absorption takes place [28]. This may be less important in species such as calves which seem less prone to hypernatraemia than infants [29].

An important factor in reversing acidosis is the restoration of normal kidney function, which itself follows restoration of circulatory volume. Nevertheless, severely acidotic animals, particularly calves, may benefit from the inclusion of bicarbonate, or preferably its pre-cursors in the formulation [30]. These and other aspects of ORS com-position have recently been reviewed [29].

Oral rehydration in calves

Oral rehydration has been most widely used in calves where adminis-tration of individual doses of oral fluid replacer is relatively easy, and where some of the principles of efficacy were established [31, 32]. Most calves find oral replacement solutions palatable, although ad-ministration by stomach tube can be an alternative where necessary, and gives similar results [32].

Oral rehydration in calves is normally recommended in association with milk deprivation for up to four feeds. This may be more than necessary, in view of the apparent digestive reserve shown at least in lambs [16]. The damage which is caused by rotavirus infection is rapidly reversible as new cells are produced which appear less suscep-tible to rotavirus infection. The normal cell turnover time in the small intestine is $3-5$ days, by which time some recovery has taken place. Therefore, milk feeding can often be reintroduced from the second feed onwards. Indeed, in the case of young pigs and single-suckled calves, it may well be impracticable to restrict milk intake at any stage, and yet results with oral rehydration under these circumstances still appear satisfactory [24]. Moreover, even relatively brief periods of food deprivation can have adverse effects on the structure of the villi [33].

Oral rehydration in pigs

Dehydration in pigs can also be conveniently treated by oral rehy-dration, and this has been shown to be effective in both rotavirus and *E. coli* induced disease [24]. Pigs will often drink oral replacement fluid when presented in a suitable container, and their intake will vary depending on need, i.e. those most requiring rehydration will consume more than those which are well hydrated. While oral re-hydration is generally safe and free from side effects, a special situation exists in hysterectomy-derived (colostrum-deprived) piglets reared in isolation. These animals have a low plasma protein concentration and so the fluid and electrolytes absorbed from the intestine pass rapidly into tissues in the presence of low plasma oncotic pressure. This can lead to fatal oedema (D. Taylor, personal communication).

The weaning period is one where oral rehydration solutions can be used to promote water absorption to minimize weight check [34, 35]. Reducing the concentration of the fluid to 150 mOsm/kg (50% of isotonic) can be effective in preventing over-consumption, and in making the use of such formulations more economically feasible.

Oral rehydration in dogs and cats

Oral rehydration fluids in dogs and cats can be useful in the treatment of dehydration due to diarrhoea, although with the notable exception of parvovirus infection, severe diarrhoeal dehydration is less common in dogs and cats than it is in young farm animals. A further use of oral rehydration is during the post-operative period, especially following conditions such as pyometra or intestinal obstruction. Here the use of oral replacement fluids can reduce the need for intravenous fluids (Chapter 11).

The palatability of oral replacement solutions for dogs and cats is such that, while the majority find them acceptable, a minority may not. It may therefore be necessary to ensure an adequate intake by dosing manually (Chapter 7).

Oral rehydration in horses

Oral rehydration in horses can be valuable in diarrhoea in foals or adults. Palatability of solutions may limit voluntary intake, in which case fluid must be given by stomach tube (Chapter 7). A mixture which may be accepted by foals when commercial solutions prove unpalatable [36] consists of NaCl 117 g, KCl 150 g, $NaHCO_3$ 168 g and K_2HPO_4 135 g: 60–90 g of this mixture is dissolved in 12 l of water and offered along with fresh water. The diluted mixture (at 90 g/12 l) contains Na 52, K 48, Cl 53 and bicarbonate 26 mmol/l; it is essentially similar to, but slightly stronger than Dalton's solution (Chapter 3). Replacement of water and electrolyte losses following prolonged exercise is conveniently achieved by oral rehydration solutions (Chapter 12).

Intravenous rehydration

The intravenous route for fluid replacement has considerable advantages in that the effect on circulatory volume is immediate, and involves no intermediate step of absorption from the intestine or from subcutaneous tissue space [37]. Unfortunately, the practical difficulties of the route make it less useful in many cases, particularly under farm conditions, although even here situations arise where intravenous fluid administration is required, and the time and effort involved can be justified [38].

The intravenous route is required when the degree of dehydration is such that the oral or subcutaneous routes are unlikely to be sufficiently rapid in their effect to save the animal. In particular, when dehydration has caused more than 8% or 9% loss of normal body weight, the peripheral circulation becomes severely restricted, and the ability to absorb fluid is likewise reduced. Oral intake by a collapsed animal is unlikely to be voluntary so that use of a stomach tube and delivery bag is the only way that the oral route can be used. The fluid still has to be passed from the rumen or stomach to the small intestine and then has to be absorbed. Both functions are unreliable in a state of collapse, which leaves the intravenous route as the only reliable alternative.

The composition of fluid lost during diarrhoea resembles that of ECF, since normally there is little tissue damage during the fluid secretion, unless either dysentery or severe desquamation of epithelia has taken place, in which case blood loss may be considerable. Some forms of diarrhoea may involve substantial enteric loss of protein. More commonly there is haemoconcentration with raised packed cell volume and serum protein concentration. Appropriate fluids will therefore contain electrolytes but no large molecular weight plasma expanding material, since this role will be carried out by the plasma protein. Similarly, whole blood is not particularly appropriate, since the cells are not required. Nevertheless, in farm animal practice, blood is a relatively convenient fluid, since it can be taken from adult animals into citrated containers and immediately infused into a collapsed recipient (Chapter 8). It has a potentially protective effect due to the immunoglobulin content. However, decisive benefit remains to be proved, and is probably offset by the relatively small volumes of blood which are infused (often less than 1 litre) in comparison with the volume needed; at a PCV of 40, 1 litre of blood provides only

600 ml of plasma. The deficit is not restricted to plasma or even ECF and, in a collapsed calf, is likely to be of the order of 4 or 5 l (10% of 40–50 kg body weight). This is roughly twice its normal plasma volume, half its ECF volume.

The aim of the fluid replacement in gastrointestinal loss is threefold:

1 To expand circulatory volume.
2 To replace electrolyte losses.
3 To correct acid–base abnormalities.

The most important of these, especially in the collapsed animal, is the expansion of circulatory volume, since this leads to restoration of kidney function, which itself is very effective in correcting acid–base imbalances. Isotonic saline is therefore often effective in reversing the symptoms of dehydration when administered in appropriate amounts but in view of the effort invested in setting up and monitoring a drip, and the likelihood of acidosis, it is more sensible to use a solution with bicarbonate or a precursor.

Solutions specifically designed for treatment of dehydration associated with gastrointestinal losses will contain alkalinizing ingredients, since diarrhoea is the most common cause and acidosis is the most common consequence. Lactate is metabolized to bicarbonate in the liver, and so indirectly acts as a source of bicarbonate, and is used for this purpose in formulations such as Darrow's and Hartmann's solutions (Chapter 3). Other precursors include acetate (Chapter 1). It has been suggested that, in the shocked animal, the conversion of lactate to bicarbonate may be impaired. In this case, severe acidosis is better treated by mixtures of precursors or specific infusions of sodium bicarbonate, which will directly treat the condition without need of intermediate metabolism. The risk of over-treatment is greatly reduced by measurement of acid–base status (Chapter 5) to allow both calculation of the likely deficit and monitoring of the response to therapy. Severe acidosis may require more bicarbonate than Hartmann's or other ECF-like solutions can provide.

Rectal administration of fluid

Enemas have been used as a means of rehydration, despite the fact that the existence of diarrhoea suggests that fluid absorption in the large intestine is already at full stretch or disrupted by the underlying pathology. It may be useful in very young pigs where the options for practical fluid therapy are extremely limited [39].

Specific examples of enteric dysfunction

Abomasal displacement/torsion in cattle

Pathophysiology

Whether the abomasum is displaced to the left or right, or whether there is torsion, the fundamental fluid and electrolyte disturbance is the same, differing only in severity [40, 41]. Vagal indigestion with abomasal impaction leads to very similar disturbances, often severe, due to reflux of abomasal fluid into the rumen [42]. The accumulation of abomasal fluid leads to metabolic alkalosis with a fall of plasma chloride. Where this fall is profound (from the normal 105 mmol/l to below 60 mmol/l) then the prognosis is particularly poor [43]. There may also be hypokalaemia caused by inappetance and exacerbated by alkalosis. Indeed, in adult cattle without diarrhoea, metabolic alkalosis is a common feature of various forms of enteric dysfunction, usually with hypokalaemia, e.g. in caecal torsion [44]. The changes tend to be mild with left displacement and most severe with abomasal torsion, in which sequestration of secretion can lead to serious dehydration.

Fluid therapy

In such cases 40−80 l of intravenous fluid may be necessary, preferably normal saline or Ringer's (bicarbonate-free) with or without additional potassium (up to 40 mmol/l). Even without measurements of plasma K^+, this concentration of potassium is likely to be safe at 5 l/hour in a 450 kg cow (less than 0.5 mmol K^+/kg/hour). A mixture of 1 : 4 isotonic KCl (1.1%) and saline (0.9%) has the composition (in mmol/l) Na 123, K 30, Cl 153. Following surgery, solutions should provide at least 50 g KCl and 50−100 g NaCl daily (as far as possible orally). The latter may alternatively be taken as *ad lib.* block salt; obviously water must be freely available and taken. Oral solutions may also include propylene glycol as an energy source [45].

Gastric dilatation/torsion complex in dogs

Pathophysiology

Acute gastric dilatation/torsion is an extremely difficult emergency to handle and mortality rates are high. Although the condition has been recorded in many breeds of dog it occurs most commonly in deep-chested breeds such as Bloodhounds, Great Danes, St Bernards, Dobermanns, Irish Setters and Wolfhounds [46]. It is not intended here to discuss the aetiology of the syndrome in detail but a variety of factors has been implicated, including the ingestion of large quantities of processed cereals and water and vigorous exercise immediately after eating [47] and an inherited predisposition has been suggested by some but not proved [48].

Whatever the initiating cause, once gas, fluid or both accumulate in the stomach, the stomach distends and may or may not then undergo torsion. Thus, it is simple progressive dilatation which is a necessary prerequisite to volvulus of the stomach. The stomach, as it distends, tends to compromise pyloric outflow by mere pressure and torsion may occur if the stomach twists on its mesenteric axis [49]. Once it is distended, the intraluminal pressure in the stomach is such that intramural ischaemia soon develops as local capillary blood flow is impaired and then gastric wall necrosis develops, usually with fatal consequences. Distension of the stomach compresses the vena cava and portal vein so that venous return to the heart is rapidly impaired and cardiac output and arterial blood pressure decrease just as quickly so that hypovolaemic shock develops very rapidly [50]. Unless corrective and supportive measures are instituted rapidly, the severe, deleterious metabolic effects of hypovolaemic shock (already discussed in Chapter 4) soon result in death.

Table 9.1 Metabolic changes in cases of gastric dilatation/torsion complex

Animal	Details	pH	P_{CO_2} (mmHg)	$[HCO_3^-]$ (mmol/l)	Base deficit (mmol/l)
German Shepherd dog	GD/T collapsed	7.416	20.7	13.3	+8.0 (acidosis)
Basset Hound	GD/T + fundic necrosis	7.225	38.8	16.0	+11.1 (acidosis)
Irish Setter	GD/T	7.275	39.2	18.2	+8.0 (acidosis)
Irish Setter	GD	7.384	51.3	30.6	−4.8 (alkalosis) (base excess)

GD/T = gastric dilatation and torsion; GD = gastric dilatation.

The metabolic changes produced by this syndrome are variable and should be assessed in the laboratory if possible (Chapter 5). Experimentally-induced gastric dilatation and torsion causes severe metabolic acidosis [50] but in clinical cases, more recent evidence has shown that this is not always so [51]. In essence, a metabolic acidosis is caused by the severe hypovolaemic shock which occurs but this tends to be partially offset by the metabolic alkalosis which results from the sequestration of H^+ ions in the fluid in the distended stomach. Theoretically, therefore, either acid−base disturbance could occur but generally speaking, most cases which are suffering from torsion and hypovolaemic shock have a metabolic acidosis in our experience (Table 9.2) while cases of dilatation alone tend to develop a metabolic alkalosis initially. The finding that an animal has a metabolic acidosis is undoubtedly a poor prognostic sign.

Fluid therapy

This needs to be instituted with great speed if the consequences of gastric dilatation/torsion are not to be fatal. In addition to instituting immediate measures to decompress the stomach, it is essential to start fluid therapy at once. A large-bore intravenous catheter must be inserted into a suitable vein and a rapid i.v infusion started. If circulatory collapse is present, then it may be necessary to cut down on to a vein in order to catheterize it. Ideally, a colloid solution should be infused initially but the nature of the fluid probably matters less than the rate at which it is being given (this should be as fast as possible, i.e. 80−100 ml/kg for the first hour). If colloid solutions are used, they should be given up to 20 ml/kg in combination with a crystalloid such as Hartmann's (in the ratio 1:3) since there is no doubt that the ECF as a whole becomes depleted in hypovolaemic shock. If no colloid is available, then lactated Ringer's may be used from the outset. The speed of infusion may be slowed once circulatory parameters start to improve (Chapters 6 and 7). If the animal is merely suffering from gastric dilatation, it is probably safer to avoid the administration of additional bicarbonate. If, however, there is also volvulus and/or the dog is exhibiting signs of shock, it is safe to assume that there is a degree of metabolic acidosis present and it is advisable to provide some 2−3 mmol bicarbonate/kg in the i.v. fluid. Hartmann's alone will only provide this at about 100 ml/kg so additional bicarbonate sources may be needed (Chapter 3).

Following rapid decompression, a transient and potentially danger-ous hyperkalaemia may occur, possibly produced as the ischaemic tissues of the stomach are suddenly reperfused and the K^+ released from damaged hypoxic cells is flushed into the general circulation. The sudden rise in plasma K^+ can be severe enough (>8 mmol/l) to induce severe cardiac arrhythmia [49] and even sudden cardiac arrest. It is therefore essential to monitor the heart closely during this period and take the appropriate measures to counteract the effect of hyper-kalaemia. Recent evidence [52, 53] indicates that 40–50% of dogs with gastric dilatation develop severe cardiac arrhythmia usually in the first 24–48 hours after admission and stabilization. The cause is unclear but probably there are many factors involved, notably myo-cardial ischaemia, hypoxia (both caused by severe shock), possibly the production of free radicals in ischaemic tissues, production of myocardial depressant factor and electrolyte imbalances. These ar-rhythmias can be refractory to therapy; if mild they need not be treated specifically though severe cases will require therapy (slow i.v. lignocaine, 2 mg/kg).

After decompression/corrective surgery, monitoring and appropri-ate i.v. fluid therapy must be continued for 24–48 hours at a rate of 50 ml/kg plus any extra required to meet any abnormal losses. Offer-ing oral fluid in this period provokes severe vomiting and should be avoided. Full return to normal oral intake may take several days and during this period there is a real danger of severe hypokalaemia (<2.5 mmol/l) which also carries with it real risks of exacerbating any cardiac arrhythmia as well as causing skeletal and smooth muscle weakness. The vicious circle of ileus producing vomiting and further hypokalaemia is obviously to be avoided. If renal function is normal following resuscitation, therefore, additional K^+ should be added to the i.v. infusion (20–30 mmol/l) in the days following surgery.

Intestinal obstruction

Obstruction of the intestinal lumen can be a simple physical block caused by a foreign body, or may result from intussusception, volvulus or a tumour. In all cases, surgical correction must be carried out urgently; fluid therapy should commence as soon as possible to correct deficits before surgery, and will continue during surgery.

The intestinal obstruction results in fluid accumulation proximal to the obstruction. Systemically, this will cause hypovolaemia, acidosis and sequestration of sodium, potassium and chloride ions in the intestine [5]. In the case of bovine intussusception, serum chloride depression is a notable feature, and is linked with a poor prognosis. In dogs and cats, vomiting may occur and hypovolaemia will lead to shock.

A functional obstruction occurs in the case of paralytic ileus. This is associated with peritonitis, or may follow handling of the small intestine during surgery. While no physical obstruction is present, the intestine no longer propels contents caudally. Accumulation of fluid with distension of the intestine aggravates the situation, and decompression is often necessary to reverse the problem. Hypokalaemia increases the risk of ileus (Chapter 2).

Fluid therapy for intestinal obstruction must primarily be by the intravenous route, although after surgery the oral route may be acceptable. The fluids used in intestinal obstruction are the same as those appropriate for diarrhoea, e.g. Hartmann's solution or other alkalinizing formulations to replace sodium, potassium, chloride and bicarbonate.

Equine colic

Pathophysiology

'Colic' in the horse is a term used to indicate abdominal pain, and as such covers a multiplicity of conditions, both surgical and medical, so that the requirements for fluid therapy vary with the pathogenesis of the causal condition. To cover all possibilities would require a book in itself, and so the following paragraphs are of necessity a simplified view of the problems.

The basic fluid requirements of the normal horse appear to be greater than those of small animals, daily intakes from 54–64 ml/kg/day having been recorded [54–56]. A 450 kg horse deprived of food and water develops a deficit of approximately 9.5 l/day [57]. This deficit is pure water loss, and is shared throughout the fluid compartments, thus allowing a large deficit to exist in the absence of severe clinical signs (see Chapter 5). In the horse deficits through water deprivation are further compensated by the large amount of water already present in the intestines which can act as a reservoir [56]. Deficits through lack of fluid intake rarely need to be taken into account in the acute surgical colic, but can become significant when water intake is denied for some time such as in choke, grass sickness, or in surgical cases which develop post-operative ileus.

In order to understand the changes in fluid and electrolyte balance which may occur in a surgical case of colic it is necessary to consider the pathophysiology of the problem [58]. The majority of conditions causing colic involve an obstruction of the intestine, and may or may not involve interference with the blood supply of the gut. These two factors both influence subsequent fluid deficits.

A simple obstruction of the small intestine rapidly results in accumulation of fluid proximal to the obstruction which causes ileus and leads to further net secretion of fluid into the gut, thus worsening the problem. Classically, it is suggested that, as in small animals, the volumes of fluid lost into the intestine in this way and the loss of bicarbonate into these fluids, results in dehydration and in acidosis [59]. However, this classical theory is no longer considered a valid explanation for the massive changes in fluid balance which occur. Although in both cases the build-up proximal to the obstruction results in fluid accumulation in the stomach, in small animals this is relieved by vomiting, and there is therefore a continuing loss of fluid from the animal. The horse does not vomit and, without intervention, the result of the fluid accumulation is rupture of the stomach, with subsequent fatal endotoxaemia and death. Experimental obstruction of the small intestine of the horse [60] has shown few changes in fluids or electrolytes for several hours until stomach rupture occurs. In clinical cases stomach tubing is used to relieve the pressure, and if this is continued for several days (as it might be in cases of grass sickness or post-operative ileus) then the fluid and bicarbonate removed must be taken into account in the design of replacement regimes, although the reserves of the horse are such that such losses have been shown to have little influence on measurable parameters of fluid balance for up to 48 hours after the onset of the obstruction [61]. In cases of simple obstruction of the large intestine, fluid is often still absorbed proximal to the block, and changes in fluid balance are even slower to occur [60, 61].

In many cases of colic which require surgery, the blood supply to the intestine is compromised. This may occur acutely, such as in cases of torsion, or more gradually as a result of pressure or of a slowly occurring thrombotic lesion. In some cases of torsion, pressure on venous outflow results in sequestration of blood or of oedema fluid into gut wall and mesentery, resulting in a rapidly developing loss of circulating volume, and in some cases death has occurred within 2 hours of onset of symptoms. More commonly, the reduced blood supply results in the integrity of the gut wall being compromised, releasing endotoxins into the circulation. The effects of endotoxaemia in the horse have been well investigated [62]. Even low doses of toxins cause a rapid rise in packed cell volume and in plasma proteins, as well as a rapid reduction in circulating volume with lowering of arterial and central venous pressures and a fall in cardiac output. The fall in circulating volume is primarily due to the sequestration of plasma fluid into the tissues as the capillary walls become more permeable. In the early stages of endotoxaemia in the horse there is a hyperglycaemia, although the animal becomes hypoglycaemic in the terminal stages [62].

Pressure on the great vessels from distended viscera can reduce cardiac output and contribute to circulatory shock, this problem becoming worse when the horse is in dorsal recumbency. Cases of simple obstruction may progress to result in necrotic gut and endotoxaemia. Conditions such as anterior enteritis may cause toxic shock in the absence of necrotic gut. There is no 'simple' case of surgical colic, and thus no easy formula for fluid requirements.

Diagnosis, pre-operative and peri-operative treatment

In the clinical situation involving the acute surgical colic the diagnosis of circulatory hypovolaemia is based on clinical examinations of heart rate, colour of mucous membranes, capillary refill, temperature of peripheral appendages; on measurement of PCV and plasma proteins [63, 64]. In endotoxic shock arterial blood pressure falls [62], and cases which are initially presented with a systolic arterial pressure of less than 60 mmHg carry a very poor prognosis [64]. Measurement of CVP tends to be less accurate as a guide to hypovolaemia in the horse than in small animals [65, 66] (Chapter 5) although its measurement may be helpful in assessing the success of therapy. In the majority of cases, the fluid has been sequestered from the circulation, and has not been lost from the animal and many of the standard signs considered to demonstrate dehydration, such as loss of skin turgor, may not be displayed [64].

There are three considerations in therapy: restoration of fluid volume, restoration of the balance of electrolytes and maintenance of acid–base balance. In the acute surgical colic case the most important factor is to restore circulating fluid volume. Classically, it has been considered that intensive fluid therapy to restore normality should be carried out before surgery, but it is now recognized that in most acute cases the situation deteriorates faster than replacement is possible, and that the priority is to remove the cause, such as the source of endotoxaemia [63]. It is obviously necessary to have an adequate circulatory volume before anaesthesia and rapid infusion of plasma or a plasma expander to reduce PCV to a maximum of 55% [63] should be carried out before induction, and further fluid replacement continued during surgery. In our experience, a surprisingly small volume of a plasma expander (5 l for a 500 kg horse) can give a significant reduction in PCV, although the effect is short lived. Further replacement is usually carried out with large volumes of ECF expanding solutions such as lactated Ringer. Volumes required are usually judged on the response to treatment, in particular by the effect on PCV, plasma proteins and on clinical indices of circulation. Although the large volumes required make over-transfusion unlikely, it must be avoided because the danger of pulmonary oedema is particularly high where toxaemia exists. Over-transfusion also results in increased secretion into the gut, counteracting the surgeon's attempts to ensure small intestinal decompression, and may indeed even contribute to post-operative ileus.

Horses with endotoxic shock usually suffer from a marked metabolic acidosis [62] but may become alkalotic in the terminal stages [63]. Lactic acidosis, as reflected by anion gap, may be a useful indicator of poor prognosis (Chapter 4). The respiratory acidosis which almost invariably occurs in anaesthetized spontaneously breathing horses may add to that induced by toxaemia, resulting in a dangerous fall in pH. Sodium bicarbonate may be given to counteract the metabolic acidosis, the total amount required being calculated by:

$$\frac{\text{BWt (kg)}}{3} \times \text{base deficit} = \text{mmol of bicarbonate required}$$

with base deficit representing the difference between normal and measured plasma bicarbonate (Chapter 5). Over-correction should be avoided (Chapter 3). Hunt [61] has shown that in most cases sodium concentrations are normal, chlorides are low, and potassium tends to be on the low side of normal; however these rarely require specific correction at this stage.

The effects of corticosteroids and of non-steroidal anti-inflammatory agents in reducing the severity of endotoxic shock in the horse have been documented [62], although both types of agent are more effective if given before shock develops; high doses of a soluble, rapidly available corticosteroid are required (Chapter 4). Suitable preparations of phenylbutazone (15−20 mg/kg) or flunixin meglumine (1.1 mg/kg) given i.v. have been recommended [62] and have the added advantage of contributing to post-operative analgesia. It must be emphasized that these drugs are given on a short term basis to avoid complications such as steroid-induced laminitis, reduced wound healing, or toxicity from the non-steroidal anti-inflammatory drugs.

Post-operative treatment

With successful surgery many patients rapidly recover gut function, can be given fluids by mouth, and create no further problems of fluid balance. However, a proportion of horses develop post-operative ileus, and these require further support. The majority of horses which develop idiopathic post-operative ileus suffer toxaemia, either initially or in the post-operative period [61]. In horses which develop ileus, PCV and plasma proteins continue to rise, further fluid therapy only giving temporary relief. Classically, the treatment of ileus is continued fluid support coupled with drainage of fluid from the intestine by stomach tube. However, drainage of the stomach does not relieve the pressure on the small intestine, and currently treatment is based on drugs, and where these fail, a second laparotomy to decompress [67]. McIlwraith [68] details a standard regime for post-operative fluid therapy, suggesting that volume is maintained with polyionic solutions, quantities being based on measurement of PCV and plasma proteins, and that electrolytes (Na, K and Cl) are monitored and disturbances corrected as necessary. If plasma proteins fall, then plasma may be given. Acid−base balance may be measured, and bicarbonate given as necessary, but it has been suggested that at this stage acidosis is usually associated with hypovolaemia and specific correction may not be required [68]. Over-administration of bicarbonate can result in hypernatraemia especially where, for example, bicarbonate is added to a standard ECF expanding solution. Where large volumes of fluid are given, peripheral oedema may occur, but in our experience pulmonary oedema is rare.

The importance of potassium levels has been the subject of much discussion. It has been suggested that low plasma potassium may increase the incidence of ileus but Hunt [61] found that in most clinical cases potassium levels were merely on the low side of normal limits, and she found no significant differences between the plasma potassium levels of horses which did or did not develop post-operative ileus.

References

1 Bywater, R.J. & Logan, E.F. (1974) The site and characteristics of intestinal water and electrolyte loss in *E. coli* induced diarrhoea in calves. *Journal of Comparative Pathology* **84**, 599−610.

2 Cummings, J.H. (1975) Absorption and secretion by the colon. *Gut* **16**, 323−9.

3 Schmall, L.M., Argenzio, R.A. & Whipp, S.C. (1983) Pathophysiologic features of swine dysentery: cyclic nucleotide-independent production of diarrhoea. *American Journal of Veterinary Research* **44**, 1309−16.

4 Hewett, G.R. (1982) Vomiting and anti-emetics in small animal practice. Pharmacologie et Toxicologie Veterinaires. INRA Publ., Paris. *Les Colloques de l'INRA 8.*

5 Twedt, D.C. & Grauer, G.F. (1982) Fluid therapy for gastrointestinal, pancreatic and hepatic disorders. *Veterinary Clinics of North America: Small Animal Practice* **12**, 463−85.

6 Chatterjee, A., Mahalanabis, D. *et al.* (1977) Evaluation of a sucrose/electrolyte solution for oral rehydration in acute infantile diarrhoea. *Lancet* **i**, 1333−5.

7 Cabello, G. (1980) Plasma cortisol and aldosterone levels in healthy and diarrhoeic calves. *British Veterinary Journal* **136**, 160−77.

8 Smith, H.W. & Halls, S. (1967) Studies on *Escherichia coli* enterotoxin. *Journal of Pathology and Bacteriology* **93**, 531−43.

9 Burgess, M.N., Bywater, R.J., Cowley, C.M., Mullan, N.A. & Newsome, P.M. (1978) Biological evaluation of a methanol soluble, heat-stable *Escherichia coli* enterotoxin in infant mice, pigs, rabbits and calves. *Infection and Immunity* **21**, 526−31.

10 Dreyfus, L.A., Jaso-Friedman, L. & Robertson, D.C. (1984) Characterisation of the mechanism of action of *Escherichia coli* heat-stable toxin. *Infection and Immunity* **44**, 493−501.

11 Hamilton, D.L., Johnson, M.R., Forsyth, G.W., Roe, W.E. & Nielsen, N.O. (1978) The effect of cholera toxin and heat-labile and heat-stable *Escherichia coli* enterotoxin on cyclic AMP concentrations in small intestinal mucosa of pig and rabbit. *Canadian Journal of Comparative Medicine* **42**, 327−31.

12 Wallis, T.S., Starkey, W.G., Stephen, J., Haddon, S.J., Osborne, M.P. & Candy, D.C.A. (1986) Enterotoxin production by *Salmonella typhimurium* strains of different virulence. *Journal of Medical Microbiology* **21**, 19−23.

13 Graham, D.Y., Sackman, J.W. & Estes, M.V. (1984) Pathogenesis of rotavirus diarrhoea. *Digestive Diseases and Sciences* **29**, 1028−35.

14 Moon, H.W. (1978) Mechanisms in the pathogenesis of diarrhoea: A review. *Journal of the American Veterinary Medical Association* **172**, 443−8.

15 Aitken, I.D. (1984) Structural and functional damage caused by viral infection of the small intestine. In: *Function and Dysfunction of the Small Intestine*, 219−46. R.M. Batt & T.L.J. Lawrence (eds). Liverpool University Press, Liverpool.

16 Ferguson, A., Paul, G. & Snodgrass, D.R. (1981) Lactose tolerance in lambs with rotaviral diarrhoea. *Gut* **22**, 114−9.

17 Porter, P. & Kenworthy, R. (1969) A study of intestinal and urinary amines in pigs in relation to weaning. *Research in Veterinary Science* **10**, 440−7.

18 Snodgrass, D.R., Terzolo, H.R., Sherwood, D., Campbell, I., Menzies, J.D. & Synge, B.A. (1986) Aetiology of diarrhoea in young calves. *Veterinary Record* **119**, 31−4.

19 Tzipori, S., Smith, M., Halpin, C., Makin, T. & Krautil, F. (1983) Intestinal changes associated with rotavirus and enterotoxigenic *Escherichia coli* infection in calves. *Veterinary Microbiology* **8**, 35−43.

20 Crane, R.K. (1969) A perspective of digestive−absorptive function. *American Journal of Clinical Nutrition* **22**, 242−9.

21 Nalin, D.R., Cash, R.A., Rahman, M. & Yunus, M.D. (1970) Effect of glycine and glucose on sodium and water absorption in patients with cholera. *Gut* **11**, 768−72.

22 Curran, P.F. (1968) Water absorption from intestine. *American Journal of Clinical Nutrition* **21**, 781−4.

23 Bywater, R.J. (1970) Some effects of *E. coli* enterotoxin on glucose and electrolyte transfer in calf small intestine. *Journal of Comparative Pathology* **80**, 565−73.

24 Bywater, R.J. & Woode, G.N. (1980) Oral fluid replacement by a glucose−glycine−electrolyte formulation in *E. coli* and rotavirus diarrhoea in pigs. *Veterinary Record* **106**, 75−8.

25 Mata, L. (1986) Cryptosporidia. *Dialogue on Diarrhoea* **27**, 1, 4.

26 Phillips, R.A. (1964) Water and electrolyte losses in cholera. *Federation Proceedings* **23**, 705−12.

27 Phillips, R.W. (1983) Oral fluid therapy: some concepts on osmolality, electrolytes and energy. *Annals de Recherches Veterinaires* **14**, 115−30.

28 Wapnir, R.A. & Lifshitz, F. (1985) Osmolality and solute concentration — their relationship with oral rehydration solution effectiveness: an experimental assessment. *Pediatric Research* **19**, 894−8.

29 Michell, A.R. (1988) Drips, drinks and drenches; what really matters in fluid therapy? *Irish Veterinary Journal* **42**, 17−22.

30 Naylor, J.M. & Forsyth, G.W. (1986) The alkalinising effects of metabolizable bases in the healthy calf. *Canadian Journal of Veterinary Research* **50**, 509−16.

31 Bywater, R.J. (1977) Evaluation of a glucose−glycine−electrolyte formulation and amoxycillin for treatment of diarrhoea in calves. *American Journal of Veterinary Research* **38**, 1983−7.

32 Cleek, J.L. & Phillips, R.W. (1981) Evaluation of a commercial preparation for oral therapy of diarrhoea in neonatal calves: administration by suckling versus intubation. *Journal of the American Veterinary Medical Association* **178**, 977−81.

33 Levin, R.J. (1984) Intestinal adaptation to dietary change as exemplified by dietary restriction studies. In: *Function and Dysfunction of the Small Intestine*, 77−93. Batt, R. & Lawrence, T. (eds). Liverpool University Press, Liverpool.

34 Bywater, R.J. (1982) Use of a glucose−glycine−electrolyte solution to stimulate water intake and absorption after early weaning. *Proceedings of the International Pig Veterinary Society Congress, Mexico City.* 257.

35 Simmons, R.D. & Keefe, T.J. (1985) Oral rehydration of neonatal calves and pigs. *Modern Veterinary Practice* **66**, 395−9.

36 Martens, R.L. & Scrutchfield, W.L. (1985) Foal diarrhoea: pathogenesis, etiology and therapy. In: *Equine Medicine and Surgery in Practice*, 200−10. Whitlock, R.H. (ed). Veterinary Learning Systems, Lawrenceville, New Jersey.

37 Watt, J.S. (1967) Fluid therapy for dehydration in calves. *Journal of the American Veterinary Medical Association* **150**, 742−50.

38 Brown, M. (1982) Simplified large animal fluid therapy. *Modern Veterinary Practice* **63**, 703−6.

39 Blackburn, P.W. (1983) Fluid therapy in pigs. *Veterinary Record* **112**, 332.

40 Hjortkjaes, R.K. & Svendsen, C.K. (1979) Right abomasal displacement in dairy cows. *Nordic Veterinary Medicine* **31**, Suppl. II, 1−28.

41 Winkler, J.K. (1977) Supportive therapy for bovine gastrointestinal strain and obstruction. *Auburn Veterinarian* (Fall), 7−11.

42 Whitlock, R.H. (1980) Bovine stomach diseases. In: *Veterinary Gastroenterology*, 410−25. Anderson, N.N. (ed). Lea & Febiger, Philadelphia.

43 Pearson, H. (1973) The treatment of disorders of the bovine abdomen. *Veterinary Record* **92**, 245−54.

44 Argenzio, R.A. & Whitlock, R.H. (1980) In: *Veterinary Gastroenterology*, 538. Anderson, N.N. (ed). Lea & Febiger, Philadelphia.

45 Gabel, A.A. & Heath, R.B. (1969) Treatment of right-sided torsion of the abomasum in cattle. *Journal of the American Veterinary Medical Association* **155**, 642−4.

46 Morgan, R.V. (1982) Acute gastric dilatation-volvulus syndrome. *Compendium of Continuing Education for the Practising Veterinarian* **8**, 677−82.

47 Van Kruiningen, H.J., Gregoire, K. & Meuten, D.J. (1974) Acute gastric dilatation: A review of comparative aspects, by species and a study in dogs and monkeys. *Journal of the American Animal Hospital Association* **10**, 294−324.

48 Stockner, P.K. (1976) Acute gastric dilatation-volvulus: a breeder's point of view. *Journal of the American Animal Hospital Association* **12**, 134−5.

49 Dann, J.R. (1976) Medical and surgical treatment of canine acute gastric dilatation. *Journal of the American Animal Hospital Association* **12**, 17−22.

50 Wingfield, W.E., Cornelius, L.M. & Deyoung, D.W. (1974) Experimental acute gastric dilatation and torsion in the dog. 1. Change in biochemical and acid base parameters. *Journal of Small Animal Practice* **15**, 41−53.

51 Wingfield, W.E., Twedt, D.C., Moore, R.W., Leib, M.S. & Wright, M. (1982) Acid base and electrolyte values in dogs with acute gastric dilatation-volvulus. *Journal of the American Veterinary Medical Association* **180**, 1070−2.

52 Leib, M.S. & Martin, R.A. (1987) Therapy of gastric dilatation-volvulus in dogs. *Compendium of Continuing Education for the Practising Veterinarian* **9**, 1155−63.

53 Van Sluijs, F.J. (1978) Gastric dilatation-volvulus in the dog. PhD Thesis, University of Utrecht, The Netherlands.

54 Tasker, J.B. (1967) Fluid and electrolyte studies in the horse. III. Intake and output of water, sodium and potassium in normal horses. *Cornell Veterinarian* **57**, 649−57.

55 Groendyk, S., English, P.B. & Abetz, I. (1988) External balance of water and electrolytes in the horse. *Equine Veterinary Journal* **20**, 189−93.

56 Waterman, A. (1977) A review of the diagnosis and treatment of fluid and electrolyte disorders in the horse. *Equine Veterinary Journal* **9**, 43−8.

57 Tasker, J.B. (1967) Fluid and electrolyte studies in the horse. IV. The effects of fasting and thirsting. *Cornell Veterinarian* **57**, 658−67.

58 Moore, J.N. & White, N.A. (1982) Acute abdominal disease. Pathophysiology and preoperative management. *Veterinary Clinics of North America: Large Animal Practice* **4**, 61−78.

59 McDonell, W.N. (1981) General anaesthesia for gastrointestinal and obstetric procedures. *Veterinary Clinics of North America: Large Animal Practice* **3**, 163−91.

60 Datt, S.C. & Usnick, E.A. (1975) Intestinal obstruction in the horse. *Cornell Veterinarian* **65**, 152−72.

61 Hunt, J.M. (1985) The pathophysiology of equine postoperative ileus. PhD Thesis, University of London.

62 Burrows, G.E. (1981) Endotoxaemic shock. *Equine Veterinary Journal* **13**, 89−94.

63 Heath, R.B. (1982) Anaesthetic management of the patient with acute abdominal disease. *Veterinary Clinics of North America: Large Animal Practice* **4**, 79−88.

64 Parry, B.W., Anderson, G.A. & Gay, C.C. (1983) Prognosis in equine colic: a comparative study of variables used to assess individual cases. *Equine Veterinary Journal* **15**, 211−15.

65 Schatzmann, U. & Battier, R. (1986/87) Some experiences with central venous (CVP) measurements in the horse. *Journal of the Association of Veterinary Anaesthetists* **14**, 109.

66 Hall, L.W. & Nigam, J.M. (1975) Measurement of central venous pressure in the horse. *Veterinary Record* **97**, 66−9.

67 Huskamp, B. (1982) The diagnosis and treatment of acute abdominal conditions in the horse. *Proceedings of the Equine Colic Research Symposium, University of Georgia,* Athens, USA.

68 McIlwraith, C.W. (1982) The acute abdominal patient, postoperative management and complications. *Veterinary Clinics of North America: Large Animal Practice* **4**, 167−83.

Chapter 10
Urinary disorders and fluid therapy

Introduction

Disorders of renal function or urine output merit particular attention in connection with fluid therapy.

1 Fluid replacement may be an important component of the management of both acute and chronic renal failure and urinary obstruction.

2 Special forms of fluid therapy, i.e. peritoneal dialysis, diuresis, provide specific methods of treating renal failure, or at least alleviating its effects.

3 Animals with renal insufficiency are more vulnerable to the fluid and electrolyte disturbances caused by ordinary disease or dysfunction, e.g. vomiting, diarrhoea, thermal stress. Not only is the kidney less able to compensate but uraemia may cause gastrointestinal dysfunction and, since it tends to suppress immune responses, there is a greater predisposition to infection. Less obvious, the effects of respiratory disease will be intensified since the renal compensation for respiratory disturbances will be restricted.

4 Perhaps most important, the usual defence against misguided or excessive fluid therapy is undermined; it is no longer enough to hope that repair of ECF volume will allow the kidney to excrete excess water and electrolytes. This problem is at its worst in acute renal failure because dehydration is an important cause yet over-hydration is one of the most important hazards.

Acute renal failure

Pathophysiological problems

Acute renal failure (ARF) involves a precipitous decline in the function of all nephrons; there is no question of unaffected nephrons compensating for the failing nephrons as in chronic renal failure (CRF). Instead, all are involved in a massive distortion of renal function, with diversion of renal blood flow away from the cortex towards the medulla and an overall reduction in renal perfusion [1–7]. Tubules may be obstructed by cell debris or precipitated proteins but this is a complication rather than an essential cause. The paradox of ARF is that despite its severe effects and (even in human medicine) its high mortality, there is the potential for complete recovery, though this may take time. CRF runs an irrevocable downward course, however slowly; there is no recovery, merely the possibility of adapting reasonably successfully to a permanent loss of renal function [8, 9].

ARF is sometimes taken to include acute decompensation of CRF, e.g. by dehydration associated with a gastrointestinal disorder. This is confusing because the underlying pathophysiology is not the same and, in particular, nephrons have been irrevocably lost: the condition arises from stresses which exceed the compensatory capacity of the surviving nephrons. Although there may be damage with ARF, e.g. acute tubular necrosis, it is essentially a functional disturbance and need not involve any lesions at all. Moreover, even where lesions occur, they may resolve especially if the basement membrane of the tubules remains intact. The proximal tubule is particularly vulnerable since known or unsuspected poisons frequently reach high concentrations at this site, either during tubular reabsorption or by being concentrated in renal cells during tubular secretion. These potential nephrotoxins include normal endogenous molecules if they become abnormal urinary constituents, e.g. haemoglobin, myoglobin, as in azoturia (Chapter 12). Clearly the risk of tubular obstruction and of high concentration of nephrotoxins is reduced by restoration of urine output. On the other hand, if fluid therapy fails to restore glomerular filtration rate (GFR) and urine output, dangerous fluid overload can develop rapidly, especially at high infusion rates.

What urine there is has a strange composition in typical ARF. Despite its small volume it is dilute but contains substantial amounts of sodium. Normally, the cause of a low urine output is dehydration and the kidney responds by concentrating urine (to conserve water) and conserving sodium (to protect ECF volume). Indeed, this is the situation in 'pre-renal failure'. With true ARF, 'intrarenal failure', the diversion of blood flow away from the cortex:

1 Impairs Na^+ conservation.
2 Impairs the excretion of K^+ and H^+.
3 Reduces GFR (and renal blood flow).

At the same time the medullary hyperaemia undermines the

production of the concentrated interstitial fluid which is the prerequisite for adequate water conservation in response to ADH (Chapter 1). Following ARF, and sometimes following urinary obstruction, 'post-renal failure', polyuria develops for a variable period. This partly reflects excretion of retained water and solute but also reflects time needed for restoration of completely normal renal function. Atypically, ARF can occur with substantial urine output [10]: at first sight this seems contradictory but it must be remembered that GFR is extremely high and even a slight mismatch with tubular reabsorption can enormously increase urine output (Chapter 1). It is thus possible to have a serious decline of GFR, impairment of tubular function, i.e. the typical features of ARF, yet an increased urine output.

A simple loss of renal function would only cause a gradual acidosis with plasma bicarbonate falling by about 2 mmol/l/day, i.e. significant acidosis would take 3–5 days to develop. Nevertheless, animals which are acutely ill with ARF may develop acidosis more rapidly as a result of enhanced catabolism [11].

Therapeutic implications

The objectives of treatment are:
1 Correction of dehydration.
2 Restoration of urine output.
3 Correction of acidosis and hyperkalaemia.
4 Reduction of azotaemia, alleviation of uraemia. This may require peritoneal dialysis (see below).

If restoration of urine output fails, the animal needs to be 'tided over', perhaps for several days, while renal function has the opportunity to recover. Maintenance solutions should be used to provide the daily water and electrolyte requirement. If over-hydration is to be avoided, voluntary and parenteral fluids should not exceed about 10 ml/kg plus all visible losses, somewhat more in young, febrile or hyperventilating animals. Body weight should be monitored and should fall by 0.5–1%/day if the animal is anorexic. The reason is that water is generated during catabolism and hydration of an anorexic animal to constant body weight implies progressive water retention, which may become serious in ARF [12, 13].

In the initial stages fluid therapy should comprise:
1 Correction of visible or suspected deficits with saline (potassium free) plus lactate or bicarbonate, e.g. a 5:1 mixture of 0.9% saline and

either $\frac{1}{6}$M (isotonic) sodium lactate or 1.5% (isotonic) sodium bicarbonate [12].

2 If urine output remains low (below 0.3 ml/kg/hour) mannitol can be used to improve renal perfusion and GFR; a test dose of 0.25–0.5 g/kg (20–25% solution) should initiate diuresis within an hour. If so, diuresis is maintained with infusions of 5–10% mannitol and electrolyte solutions as in **1**. Urine output is monitored and losses replaced [12–14]. Alternatively, hypertonic glucose may initiate diuresis [15, 16, 26], but although there are no direct comparisons, there is less evidence for beneficial effects on renal function than with mannitol [12]; nevertheless the question remains open [27].

3 If osmotic diuresis fails, frusemide or another loop diuretic provides an alternative means of restoring output (initial dose 2–4 mg/kg, i.v.). Losses should be replaced with electrolyte solutions as in **1**.

The need to monitor urine output justifies the use of a urinary catheter but meticulous precautions are needed to minimize the risk of infection since animals with ARF are more susceptible.

Hyperkalaemia may require specific treatment, as indicated by plasma levels above 6 mmol/l, or ECG changes (bradycardia, peaked or biphasic T-waves, depressed P-waves, widened QRS). As discussed in Chapter 2, its effects can be countered by 10% calcium gluconate at 0.5–1 ml/kg, or corrected by:

1 Treatment of acidosis (1 mmol of bicarbonate/kg if no measurements available).

2 Hypertonic glucose (20–30%, 4 ml/kg), with or without insulin (0.5 units/kg) [12–14]. This works by promoting cellular uptake of K^+, rather than through osmotic diuresis.

Chronic renal failure

Pathophysiological problems

CRF involves a balance between progressive loss of nephrons, with an overall decline in GFR, and compensatory responses in surviving nephrons, notably hyperperfusion and an increase in their individual GFR [9]. The tubules of these intact surviving nephrons are subjected to much higher flow rates and solute loads and some of their compensatory capacity is already engaged at rest. They are unlikely to be able to achieve extremes of urine composition and, in this sense, the kidneys become 'inflexible', i.e. less responsive to everyday stresses such as changes in dietary intake, fluid intake, or even mild pathological losses during diarrhoea, vomiting, bleeding, fever, high environmental temperature, etc. On the other hand, adaptive responses allow surviving nephrons to become much more efficient at secreting potassium so that hyperkalaemia is only a problem in advanced cases or those with other disturbances. Advanced CRF causes metabolic acidosis for two reasons: initially failure of H^+ secretion and bicarbonate retention (normal anion gap). Excretion of H^+ is restricted by reduced availability of urinary buffers. Finally, acid anions are retained and anion gap increases [3]. Dogs with CRF have an unusual ability to resist the development of acidosis due to a compensatory increase in renal bicarbonate retention; the risk of bone damage is thus diminished [12]. Nevertheless, the main cause of bone damage in renal failure is impaired calcium absorption resulting from a reduction in the activation of vitamin D and leading to increased secretion of parathyroid hormone (PTH). This is reinforced by hyperphosphataemia, because CRF restricts the ability of the kidneys to excrete the phosphate liberated from bone minerals alongside calcium (PTH causes renal Ca^{++} retention but normally promotes phosphate excretion, until GFR is low) [9].

Some dogs have specific defects in proximal or distal tubular function leading to renal tubular acidosis (e.g. Fanconi syndrome) [12]. They require substantial quantities of bicarbonate to correct their metabolic acidosis and if possible this should be mixed into food [16].

The kidneys confront particular problems in maintaining sodium balance during CRF:

1 There are fewer nephrons to excrete the daily excess of ingested Na^+; a greater proportion of filtered Na^+ therefore needs to be excreted. This may be helped by an increased concentration of natriuretic hormones, notably circulating inhibitors of sodium transport which increase in concentration during uraemia, especially if sodium intake is high [9].

2 Despite this increase in the *proportion* of Na^+ excreted, the *absolute* amount reabsorbed by each surviving nephron is also increased, because its GFR is substantially increased. Were this not so, the increase in GFR in these intact nephrons would rapidly cause Na^+ depletion

3 The likelihood of achieving zero sodium concentration in urine, when necessary (i.e. in response to aldosterone during ECF volume depletion) is greatly diminished by the increased flow rate in surviving nephrons and the consequent reduction in time for complete reabsorption.

There are thus sound reasons to predict that CRF may lead to sodium loss or sodium retention according to the individual patient and its diet. The question is, which matters more — and which is most likely? There is no doubt that sodium depletion, dehydration, loss of circulating volume (e.g. haemorrhage) can seriously decompensate a failing kidney and produce a uraemic crisis, 'acute on chronic'.

The main risk of sodium retention is that it may exacerbate hypertension. While it is true that hypertension in dogs is probably under-diagnosed, it also seems likely that they are peculiarly resistant to it, even when they have CRF [17]. Moreover, even with advanced CRF, the kidney remains able to preserve sodium balance provided any change in intake (or onset of loss) is sufficiently *gradual*. On balance, therefore, salt restriction is hard to justify but salt loading is unnecessary and may be risky. Dehydration and salt loss should certainly be treated, initially by oral rehydration unless vomiting precludes it or the deficits are too severe. The idea that this is contraindicated because of a need for salt restriction is absurd. When parenteral therapy is needed, care must be taken to avoid excessive infusion rates because uraemia can impair cardiac function and affect the pulmonary circulation; both will predispose to pulmonary oedema [18].

Hyponatraemia

Hyponatraemia may be a problem in oliguric patients allowed too much fluid, or as a result of salt wasting during the diuresis which follows ARF or urinary obstruction, or in a minority of animals with CRF which have urinary salt wasting and polydipsia [15]. This poses the unusual problem of needing to correct plasma sodium concentration while avoiding excessive ECF expansion. It is one of the few justifications in veterinary fluid therapy for the use of hypertonic saline. One litre of 5% saline (855 mmol/l) has 710 mmol/l of excess Na^+, assuming a normal ECF concentration of 145 mmol/l.

The effect of giving 1 ml/kg of hypertonic saline is as follows:

1 ml/kg body weight
= 1 ml/0.6 l of total body water (60% body weight)
= 0.710 mmol of extra Na^+/0.6 l of total body water

i.e. it raises ECF [Na$^+$] by 1.2 mmol/l.

Note that although Na$^+$ is restricted to ECF, the effect of *additional* Na$^+$ is *as if* it were distributed *throughout* the body water — because although they contain different solutes, ECF and ICF must change equally in osmotic concentration as water redistributes between them until they do. The useful rule of thumb is that

5% saline @ 1 ml/kg raises plasma Na$^+$ by 1.2 mmol/l.

Since symptomatic hyponatraemia probably involves a fall of 15 mmol/l or more, correction requires doses of the order of 15 ml/kg, i.e. 300 ml in a 20 kg dog. To get the same effect with 'normal saline' would require about 1.7 l — a considerable difference when volume overload is a potential problem. In fact one would use about half the suggested dose of hypertonic saline in order to half correct the disturbance initially and avoid violent changes in plasma Na$^+$. Both with onset and treatment of disturbances of plasma Na$^+$ concentration, speed of change rather than magnitude correlates with severity of effect.

Therapeutic implications

1 It is essential to correct any ECF volume depletion urgently.
2 The polydipsia of CRF is secondary to polyuria resulting from inability to concentrate the urine. Inadequate drinking will lead to dehydration with the risk of hypernatraemia. In this case parenteral provision of water as 5% glucose or as a maintenance solution becomes necessary.
3 It is advisable to provide bicarbonate, e.g. via Hartmann's solution, if parenteral fluids are used. This will not raise plasma bicarbonate above normal, and will help to correct any underlying acidosis. Additional bicarbonate sources may be needed if acidosis is more severe.
4 Hartmann's solution is not contraindicated despite the presence of K$^+$; it is no more than contained in plasma and if acidosis is improved, K$^+$ entry to cells may otherwise cause hypokalaemia [19]. It must be emphasized that, except during acute decompensation or advanced failure, hyperkalaemia is not a predominant feature of CRF and anorexia readily predisposes to hypokalaemia. The fact that Hartmann's solution contains some Ca^{++} is helpful since the acidosis which accompanies uraemia has one beneficial effect; it tends to liberate some of the protein-bound calcium in plasma and offset the effect of any

fall in Ca^{++} due to CRF. This benefit is lost once the acidosis improves.

5 The metabolic disturbances of uraemia, combined with anorexia, could make animals with CRF candidates for parenteral nutrition. Unless it is to tide them over a short term crisis this scarcely seems justifiable, especially since the sustained use of nutrient fluids carries the risk of phlebitis and infection and uraemia tends to be immuno-suppressive. There is probably more justification for parenteral nutrition in extended ARF — but there is the risk of infection (Chapter 12).

Nephrotic syndrome

Pathophysiological problems

Nephrotic syndrome is the result of glomerular damage severe enough to cause heavy proteinuria, leading to a fall of plasma albumin concentration and the development of oedema [1, 2]. There may also be a substantial rise in blood lipids [20] and, by 'diluting' plasma with a non-aqueous component, this may lead to a false or exaggerated hyponatraemia (sodium being restricted to the aqueous component) [21].

Since interstitial fluid is a large compartment, its pathological expansion (from plasma) can only occur if the kidney keeps 'topping up' plasma volume, i.e. retaining sodium and water. Paradoxically, therefore, the mechanisms regulating sodium and water balance behave as if plasma volume were reduced, despite the visible results of ECF expansion. Indeed, plasma volume may genuinely be subnormal, and plasma sodium concentration may genuinely fall, as in other forms of volume depletion [11, 21–22]. The fall in plasma protein concentration will almost inevitably depress total calcium but it should be emphasized that free, ionized calcium is likely to be normal and so, therefore, is the animal where calcium is concerned.

Nephrotic syndrome may or may not be accompanied by azotaemia [23] (biochemical signs of nitrogenous end product retention) or uraemia (the equivalent clinical signs). The condition poses difficult contradictions [16]:

1 The loss of urinary protein increases protein requirement — but uraemia requires protein restriction.

2 Despite the excess ECF volume, plasma volume may be subnormal

or, certainly, vulnerable to any cause of hypovolaemia. Thus, salt restriction and/or the use of diuretics are logical ways of reducing the oedema but, especially in a uraemic animal, they may lead to hypovolaemia, reduced GFR, and an acute crisis in renal function. Equally, the use of albumin to protect plasma volume may also increase nitrogen load in a uraemic animal [12].

3 Clearly, hypovolaemia must be avoided but so must circulatory overload and expansion of ECF — the latter is already one of the main problems of nephrotic syndrome. Moreover, the general tendency towards oedema means that the risk of pulmonary oedema will be greater than in normal animals.

4 If acidosis is severe enough to need treatment, e.g. if uraemia is prominent, there is a contradiction between provision of bicarbonate (or its precursors) and restriction of sodium. Use of calcium lactate to provide some of the bicarbonate reduces this problem [12, 24].

Therapeutic implications

1 Diuresis must not be too fast or too intense because if it outstrips the speed of mobilization of oedema fluid (including ascitic fluid) it will cause hypovolaemia [22].

2 Since it is only plasma volume which is liable to be depleted in nephrotic syndrome, a strong logical justification points to the use of colloids rather than crystalloids [25]. They may be less effectively retained, however, due to the altered glomerular permeability.

3 If a nephrotic syndrome, or its treatment, is accompanied by a uraemic crisis, repair of any hypovolaemia becomes vital, but it is even more important than usual to avoid excessive infusion rates, in view of the risk of pulmonary oedema.

Diuresis and peritoneal dialysis

Two more specific forms of fluid therapy are now considered briefly: the use of diuresis and fluid replacement or of peritoneal dialysis to substitute for renal function.

Diuresis and fluid replacement

This simply involves increasing fluid turnover and, therefore, the excretion of nitrogenous waste. It is not improving renal function, i.e.

restoring GFR. The object of the diuresis is to remove products which are normally excreted, not to dehydrate the patient, hence the importance of matching fluid replacement. A typical approach is to alternate 40–50 ml/kg of Hartmann's solution with 40–50 ml/kg of 5% dextrose at 1 ml/kg/minute, i.e. 800 ml at 20 ml/minute for a 20 kg dog, taking 40 minutes [15, 25]. This is well above the rate of glucose infusion to exceed the renal threshold of the dog (about 0.5 g/kg/hour) [13] and should provoke a good diuresis. The bladder should be emptied and kept catheterized in order to confirm that by the time half the infusion has been given, urine output is at least 1 ml/10 kg body weight; if not, the infusion should be stopped.

Peritoneal dialysis [28–30]

This involves the use of the peritoneum as a dialysing membrane to permit the removal of waste products from plasma. The object is to place sterile fluid in the abdomen, at a temperature allowing efficient exchange, and to remove it after a suitable period for equilibration. The process is repeated through several cycles, particularly because it may be difficult to retrieve all the fluid from the initial exchange (dead space effect). Only the removal of the peritoneal infusion actually benefits the animal. Since the object is to remove *abnormal* constituents of plasma it is important that normal constituents, notably sodium, chloride and bicarbonate, are at plasma-like concentration. Potassium is omitted because peritoneal dialysis is usually employed to treat ARF or acute decompensation and in both cases hyperkalaemia is likely. The solution needs to be slightly hypertonic to normal plasma, because the osmolarity of plasma is higher in uraemic animals and unless the solution is more concentrated it will tend to be absorbed into circulation. This defeats the object, i.e. retrieving the equilibrated fluid and thus removing some of the solutes normally excreted in urine. The additional osmoles in dialysis fluid are usually provided in the form of glucose (Table 10.1).

Urinary obstruction: post-renal failure

Pathophysiological problems

Post-renal failure describes the development of azotaemia or uraemia as a result of factors beyond the kidney. The main problems are thus

Table 10.1 Typical formulation for peritoneal dialysis

		mmol/l	
Na		140	
K		0	
Ca		2.5	
Mg		0.8	
Cl		100	
Lactate		45	(often acetate)
Dextrose monohydrate (g/l)		15	
Total osmolality		364	

urine retention and its consequences, as a result of urinary obstruction or bladder dysfunction, and in the extreme cases the consequences of a ruptured bladder. This presents the combined potential hazards of chemically induced peritonitis, uraemia due to rapid absorption of urinary contents, and of infection. The adverse effects of urinary obstruction are not necessarily resolved by relief of the obstruction. Depending whether the obstruction was total or partial, unilateral or bilateral, acute or chronic, there may be a profound 'post-obstructive diuresis' which may take some days or even longer to subside completely [2, 12]. During this period it is important that the animal is able to make good its losses, by eating and drinking, and that any development of dehydration is speedily identified and treated. In contrast with the hyperkalaemia seen during obstruction, post-obstructive diuresis may cause hypokalaemia through excessive urinary losses. Until renal function returns to normal, the animal remains more vulnerable to disturbances associated with other causes of dehydration. Weight changes are an important component of monitoring because in the early stages of diuresis some of the losses may be appropriate, i.e. excretion of retained solutes, but the sustained losses are due to defects in renal function, including tubular reabsorption of sodium and water.

Therapeutic implications

1 Appropriate fluid therapy may make the difference between a successful and an unsuccessful outcome in cases of urinary obstruction [16, 31]. While obstruction persists, the priority is to treat hyperkalaemia and acidosis. Treatment of dehydration is also important because even if no urine is produced, there is probably little intake of food or water and insensible losses continue; vomiting is also likely. Particularly with a ruptured bladder there may be shock so that despite the absence of external losses, volume replacement is important.

2 It is desirable to monitor both plasma K^+ and acid—base status; both are now feasible within the range of instruments appropriate to a practice laboratory (Chapter 5). The acidosis can be helped by Hartmann's solution but it only contains as much bicarbonate (precursor) as plasma and its K is initially undesirable (though plasma K is likely to fall as acidosis improves). Moreover, the usual argument that restoration of ECF volume will allow the kidney to restore plasma pH does not apply in urinary obstruction. A mixture of 50 : 50 isotonic saline and dextrose has the advantage of absence of potassium and presence of glucose, both of which help to reverse hyperkalaemia. Bicarbonate or a precursor should be added according to severity of acidosis.

3 While an animal is neither eating nor drinking adequately it is essential to provide maintenance requirements. For a cat, 60—80 ml/kg/ day is appropriate and could be Hartmann's solution i.v. or s.c. [16, 26]. Alternatively, a standard maintenance solution can be used intravenously — these usually contain more K^+ and are therefore less suitable while obstruction persists but more suitable subsequently. Indeed, once obstruction is relieved, hypokalaemia may become severe and necessitate solutions containing 20—30 mmol/l K^+ (at rates not to exceed 0.5 mmol/kg/hour) [12, 14]

4 One particularly important reason for worrying about hypokalaemia during post-obstructive diuresis is that it is liable to cause smooth muscle ileus (including possible atony of the bladder). The safest route for replacement of K^+ deficits is always oral and both for this reason, and to combat dehydration and volume depletion resulting from diuresis, early restoration of food and water intake is desirable. Oral rehydration solutions may be useful at this stage.

5 Although it is peripheral to fluid therapy, it is worth emphasizing that urinary obstruction tends to cause metabolic acidosis and that this can be severe; any idea of using urinary acidifiers in the immediate aftermath (to prevent urolithiasis) is inappropriate since these work essentially by causing a metabolic acidosis [14, 32].

6 As recovery from obstruction progresses, diuresis may result from overuse of fluids or from incomplete recovery of renal function. During this period restoration of voluntary eating and drinking is important, together with 'tapering off' rather than abrupt withdrawal of fluid support; monitoring of hydration is important until clinical recovery is complete.

Traumatic post-renal uraemic syndrome in small animals

Blunt trauma (due to a road traffic accident) is frequently associated with damage to the lower urinary tract. Where this interferes with normal excretion of urine it requires prompt attention; however the clinician should not be too eager to resort to immediate anaesthesia and surgery before stabilizing the animal's metabolic condition. Selcer [33] recorded a 16% incidence of urinary tract damage associated with pelvic trauma in 100 dogs and 7% of these were urinary bladder ruptures and 5% urethral ruptures. He found no sex predisposition for damage to the urinary tract. Most interestingly no obvious clinical signs were present in one-third of these cases with the females being less likely to exhibit signs than the males. The finding offers a possible explanation of the generally accepted belief that females are less likely to sustain urinary tract injury than male dogs [34]. The lack of clinical signs also serves to emphasize the importance of making a positive effort to check the integrity of the urinary tract following abdominal or pelvic trauma.

Rupture of the bladder is the commonest type of injury encountered but ureteric avulsion and intraperitoneal rupture of the urethra will produce similar clinical signs. Bladder rupture is most likely when the bladder is full at the time of the accident and most tears occur at the fundus [35]. Clinical signs develop within 24–36 hours but, because the animals frequently have concurrent fractures of hindlimbs and/or pelvis, the clinician may not attribute the pain and deteriorating condition of the animal to urinary tract damage. It is important to emphasize at this point that the ability to void urine is no indication that the bladder is intact and radiography is essential in diagnosing/ruling out urinary tract damage.

Abdominal tenderness is probably the most common clinical sign encountered in such cases; progressive abdominal distension, increasing dullness, vomiting and pyrexia soon follow. Experimentally induced bladder trauma resulted in death within 90 hours (mean survival time 65 hours) [36]. Clinical cases which have been subjected to severe blunt trauma are usually dead within 3 days.

Intraperitoneal rupture of the urethra is the second most common serious urinary tract injury following pelvic trauma and the clinical and metabolic changes which occur are identical to those encountered following vesical rupture.

Retroperitoneal urethral rupture, however, is not characterized by such dramatic and rapidly fatal consequences. It occurs quite often in cats following blunt trauma to the perineal region, when it is associated with sacrococcygeal injuries. Leakage of sterile urine is relatively harmless for 24−36 hours but, if undetected, cellulitis and ultimately extensive skin sloughing will occur.

Urinary obstruction in horses (foals)

Uroperitoneum in the adult horse is rare and usually associated with a ruptured bladder, secondary to complete urethral obstruction by calculi. Rupture of the bladder, however, is seen sporadically in foals, and has been attributed to extreme pressures applied to a distended bladder at the time of parturition. This hypothesis is supported by the higher incidence in male foals, where the long narrow urethra favours rupture of the bladder rather than its emptying. However, the condition occasionally occurs in females, thus suggesting that some other mechanism must also be involved. Evidence at surgery confirms that most cases are indeed traumatic in origin, but rarely congenital defects have been suspected [37]. The site of rupture can vary; some authors believe that the rupture occurs most frequently in the dorsal wall of the bladder [38] but others [39] have recorded five out of 22 cases where the tear was in the ventral bladder. They also recorded several cases where the urachus was ruptured and these animals presented with signs indistinguishable from those of rupture of the bladder.

Affected foals become progressively dull following birth and unless diagnosed are typically presented at the age of 4−5 days often in a moribund condition. Complete anuria is unusual and this continued ability to void small quantities of urine often leads to cases of ruptured bladder being confused with cases of retained meconium. However, the latter present with marked faecal tenesmus and a characteristic stance with arching of the back, and suffer colic. In addition, dysuric foals generally have marked abdominal distension, with a palpable fluid wave. Abdominocentesis should confirm the presence of uroperitoneum. The principles of treatment remain the same as in small animals.

Urinary obstruction in ruminants

Urolithiasis is the commonest cause of rupture of the bladder and/or urethra in cattle and sheep. It is therefore a condition which predominantly occurs in young castrated male animals being fed a high concentrate ration, but can also occur in older entire males when it may be associated with pyelonephritis and calculi in the renal pelvis. There may be a breed predisposition in sheep (Texel, Blackface) reflecting differences in urinary versus faecal phosphate excretion [41]. Obstruction of the urethra by calculi is usually complete and these animals are observed straining, unsuccessfully, to urinate. The reason for the high incidence of this disease in castrated males is the small diameter of the urethra, especially at the sigmoid flexure, in cattle and sheep and additionally at the vermiform appendage in sheep, the two sites where obstruction occurs. Rupture of the urethra and, subsequently, the bladder may also be a consequence of careless application of a Burdizzo at the time of castration.

Affected animals become dull, with obvious pain and abdominal distension and on abdominal or rectal palpation a tense, distended bladder can be felt. If not diagnosed early the increased intravesical pressure eventually leads to bladder rupture, although the severe metabolic changes which occur sometimes lead to the animal's demise before the bladder ruptures. If left untreated these animals frequently survive 7−10 days before dying; again, the principles of treatment are the same as in small animals.

Laboratory findings in cases of rupture of the urinary bladder or intraperitoneal urethra

Animals quickly become dehydrated with an elevated haematocrit and serum urea levels. Serum creatinine levels also become elevated and this is probably a more reliable indicator than urea levels since the latter can be affected by extra-renal factors including gastrointestinal haemorrhage. A useful diagnostic test is to compare urea and creatinine levels in the blood and the intraperitoneal fluid; creatinine particularly is likely to be present in high concentrations when free urine is present in the peritoneum.

Hyponatraemia, hypochloraemia and hyperkalaemia are all consistent findings in clinical cases of uroperitoneum although in experimentally induced rupture of the bladder in dogs [36] it was found that hyperkalaemia did not develop until some 45 hours after rupture.

In foals, because their dietary intake (mare's milk) is low in sodium and high in potassium, these changes are likely to be even more marked and rapid in onset.

Acid—base changes

Experimentally induced rupture of the bladder in dogs was not characterized by marked acid—base changes until the animals were terminally ill, according to Burrow and Bovee [36]. Their explanation for the absence of a metabolic acidosis in these animals was that severe vomiting, by causing a loss of H^+ and Cl^- ions, resulted in an alkalosis which counteracted the retention of H^+ ions occurring as a result of the uroperitoneum. Our experience of cases of ruptured bladder in all species has not confirmed their findings. In a series of cases of uroperitoneum, hyperkalaemia and a marked metabolic acidosis have been consistent laboratory findings, and in general the severity of the hyperkalaemia and the acidosis have been closely correlated (Table 10.2). One exception to this finding was a case of complete urethral obstruction in a Golden Retriever (Table 10.3). This lesion had been misdiagnosed and the animal had been treated for 5 days with purgatives and was presented moribund, having been vomiting incessantly since the onset of illness. On first examination

Table 10.2 Haematological findings in dogs with rupture of the bladder and intraperitoneal urethra

Breed	Flat coat Retriever	Collie	Spaniel	CKC Spaniel
Sex	Male	Female	Male	Female
Problem	Ruptured bladder	Ruptured bladder	Ruptured urethra	Ruptured urethra
PCV %	44.0	NM	42.0	22.5
TSP g/dl	NM	NM	7.4	4.46
Urea mmol/l	40.0	NM	21.2	61.5
K^+ mmol/l	7.1	NM (4.89 3 days earlier)	7.4	4.74
pHV	7.188	7.211	7.322	7.149
P_{CO_2}V	34.0	29.3	27.7	34.5
[HCO_3] mmol/l	13.0	11.7	14.3	12.0
Base deficit	+13.8	+14.8	+9.7	+16.2

NM = not measured.

Table 10.3 Haematological findings in cases of urethral obstruction — dogs and cats

Species/breed	Cat	Cat	Sealyham	Golden Retriever	
Sex	Male	Male	Male	Male	
Problem	FUS	FUS	Calculi	Calculi + excessive vomiting	
				Initial	*After fluids* (saline)
PCV %	—	—	51.0	44.5	
Urea mmol/l	43.2	56.8	26.7	44.6	
K$^+$ mmol/l	9.1	8.1	3.38	8.9	
pHV	7.10	7.144	7.259	7.513	7.329
P_{CO_2}V	35.0	37.1	31.4	42.3	12.6
[HCO$_3^-$]	11.7	12.7	14.0	33.9	7.0
Base deficit	+16.8	+15.8	+11.7	10.9	+15.5

he was found to be suffering from a severe metabolic alkalosis, associated unusually with a high serum potassium. After fluid therapy to correct the alkalosis, but before relief of the obstruction, a second examination revealed the metabolic acidosis which had previously been masked (Table 10.3). We find that foals with uroperitoneum also develop a metabolic acidosis but Richardson and Kohn [39] in reviewing 22 cases suggest that the changes may not always be severe.

Therapy for post-renal uraemia

The gravest risk for cases of uroperitoneum or complete urethral obstruction is the immediate induction of general anaesthesia in a misguided attempt to relieve the obstruction or repair the defect immediately.

There are two aspects of the animal's condition which must be borne in mind in relation to anaesthesia. Firstly, the presence of a large volume of fluid, either free or within a grossly distended bladder, greatly increases intra-abdominal pressure, splitting the diaphragm and effectively limiting respiratory excursions. The increased pressure also adversely affects cardiovascular function by increasing peripheral resistance. It cannot be sensible to anaesthetize any animal without first slowly draining the accumulated urine to reduce the degree of cardiopulmonary compromise.

Secondly, the likely presence of hyperkalaemia and metabolic acidosis compounds the risk of severe cardiac irregularities and even cardiac arrest under anaesthesia. High serum potassium levels (> 8 mmol/l) are severely cardiotoxic producing marked dysrhythmias, and hyperkalaemia should always be suspected if the animal has a bradycardia. Electrocardiographic changes typically induced by hyper-kalaemia [42] include:

Peaking of the T-wave

Decreased amplitude of the P-wave

Prolonged P—R interval

Increased duration of the QRS complex

Shortened Q—T interval.

Figure 10.1 shows an ECG trace from a dog suffering from a ruptured bladder of 5 days' duration following a road traffic accident.

Severe atrioventricular conduction disturbances are likely leading to third degree A—V block, premature ventricular contractions and even ventricular fibrillation and cardiac arrest. The superimposition of a cardiotoxic drug, such as halothane, and hypercarbia, produced by the respiratory depression caused by anaesthesia, makes the pro-gression to severe and possibly fatal cardiac dysrhythmias even more likely.

Hyponatraemia alone does not affect cardiac function but will potentiate the effects of hyperkalaemia [40].

Correction of metabolic and electrolyte disturbances

The main aim of fluid therapy is to counteract the metabolic acidosis, correct the hyperkalaemia and treat the dehydration. The *fluid of choice* is a combination of normal saline (0.9%) and dextrose (5%) together with sodium bicarbonate (4.2% or 5%) to treat the metabolic acidosis.

The *volume* of fluid required depends on the severity of the signs. A volume approximately equal to 5% of the body weight in kg can be given in mild cases of short duration, and up to 10—12% in severe cases. Fluid therapy should be continued until the animal's condition has stabilized sufficiently to allow anaesthesia to be induced safely for the correction of the problem.

In cases of ruptured bladder it is sensible to catheterize the bladder so that any urine that is being produced is drained immediately. In cases of urethral obstruction direct drainage of a grossly distended bladder via a needle or catheter may be indicated.

It is essential *to treat the hyperkalaemia* which is present. Mild to moderate cases (5—7 mmol/l) are usually corrected merely by the dilutional effect of giving fluids, combined with the correction of the

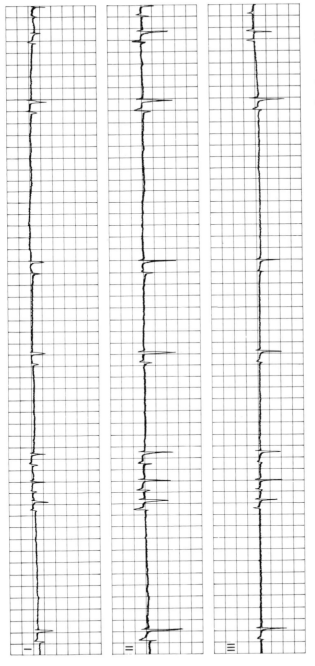

Fig. 10.1 ECG trace from a labrador suffering from fractured pelvis and ruptured bladder of 5 days duration. Note the absence of P-waves and bradycardia.

metabolic acidosis and the administration of dextrose which promotes the intracellular transfer of potassium. Severe cases (< 8 mmol/l) suffering from cardiac arrhythmias may need to be treated, additionally, by the slow intravenous injection of 10% calcium gluconate (0.5−1 ml/kg) in order to antagonize the effects of the potassium ions on the heart directly. In addition to drainage of urine from the peritoneal cavity, peritoneal lavage/dialysis with several litres of normal saline will also help to lower plasma K^+ and urea levels very quickly in severely compromised animals.

Ideally, *correction of acid−base imbalance* should be titrated according to the bicarbonate levels found in the blood. However, in the absence of facilities for measuring blood gases or total CO_2, experience has shown that these animals usually have a base deficit of at least 10 mmol/l. Thus, the administration of 2−3 mmol/kg of sodium bicarbonate is entirely safe provided it is not too fast. Normal saline (0.9%) is usually sufficient to correct the hyponatraemia except that in foals the sodium deficit may be so severe that *hypertonic* (5%) saline may be indicated, as otherwise over-hydration might occur [39].

Fluid administration should be continued after surgical correction of the problem, especially if it was one of urethral obstruction. Subcutaneous fluids may be substituted for intravenous fluids provided they are isotonic and contain adequate Na^+ but the likelihood of post-obstructive diuresis means that fluid requirements are increased for 24−48 hours. Since hypokalaemia (< 3.0 mmol/l) may also develop immediately after the relief of an obstruction, especially if the animal remains anorexic and potassium-free fluids have been used, the maintenance fluid should be changed to Hartmann's rather than to 0.9% saline once surgery has been carried out or the obstruction relieved.

References

1 Michell, A.R. (1980) The kidney: regulation and disturbances of body fluids. In: *Physiological Basis of Small Animal Medicine*, 71−126. Yoxall, A.T. & Hird, J.F.R. (eds). Blackwell Scientific Publications, Oxford.

2 Michell, A.R. (1983) Abnormalities of renal function. In: *Veterinary Nephrology*, 189−210. Hall, L.W. (ed). Heinemann, London.

3 Walmsley, R.N. & Guerin, M.D. (1984) In: *Disorders of Fluid and Electrolyte Balance*, 171−205. Wright, Bristol.

4 Rainford, D.J. (1982) Acute renal failure. In: *Treatment of Renal Failure*, 1−32. Castro, J.E. (ed). MTP Press, Lancaster.

5 Brenner, B.M. & Lazarus, J.M. (1988) *Acute Renal Failure* (2nd edn), 3–173. Churchill Livingstone, New York.

6 Ross, L.A. (1986) Feline renal failure. In: *Nephrology and Urology*, 109–36. Breitschwerdt, E.B. (ed). Churchill Livingstone, New York.

7 Senior, D.F. (1983) Acute renal failure in the dog. *Journal of the American Animal Hospital Association* **19**, 837–45.

8 Bovee, K.C. (1988) Management of chronic renal failure. In: *Renal Disease in Dogs and Cats*, 145–60. Michell, A.R. (ed). Blackwell Scientific Publications, Oxford.

9 Michell, A.R. (1988) Renal function, renal damage and renal failure. In: *Renal Disease in Dogs and Cats*, 5–29. Michell, A.R. (ed). Blackwell Scientific Publications, Oxford.

10 Low, D.G. & Cowgill, L.D. (1983) Emergency management of the acute uremic crisis. In: *Current Veterinary Therapy VIII*, 981–9. Kirk, R.W. (ed). W.B. Saunders, Philadelphia.

11 Carpenter, B. & Rault, R. (1985) Parenchymal disease and renal failure. In: *Disorders of Fluid and Electrolyte Balance*, 161–88. Puschett, J.B. (ed). Churchill Livingstone, New York.

12 Bovee, K.C. (1984) *Canine Nephrology*, 405–38, 707–21. Harwal, USA.

13 Michell, A.R. (1979) The pathophysiological basis of fluid therapy and some specific applications to medical conditions in small animals. *Veterinary Record* **104**, 542–8; 572–5.

14 Chew, D.J. & Di Bartola, S.P. (1986) *Manual of Small Animal Nephrology and Urology*, 79–146, 197–226. Churchill Livingstone, New York.

15 Lage, A.L. (1982) Fluid therapy for renal disorders. *Veterinary Clinics of North America: Small Animal Practice* **12**, 487–99.

16 Lewis, L.D., Morris, M.L. & Hand, M.S. (1987) *Small Animal Clinical Nutrition III*, 8:42–7; 9:20–31; 10:19–32. Mark Morris Associates, Topeka.

17 Michell, A.R. (1989) Salt intake, animal health and hypertension. In: *Recent Advances in Dog and Cat Nutrition*. Rivers, J. & Burger, I. (eds). Cambridge University Press, Cambridge. In Press.

18 Thier, S.O. (1983) Organ systems effects of chronic renal failure. In: *Pathophysiology*, 915–20. Smith, L.H. & Thier, S.O. (eds). W.B. Saunders, Philadelphia.

19 Cornelius, L.M. (1983) Fluid therapy in the uraemic patient. In: *Current Veterinary Therapy VIII*, 989–94. Kirk, R.W. (ed). W.B. Saunders, Philadelphia.

20 Osborne, C.A., Finco, D.R. & Low, D.G. (1984) Pathophysiology of renal disease, renal failure and uraemia. In: *Veterinary Internal Medicine*, 2nd edn. 1733–92. Ettinger, S.J. (ed). W.B. Saunders, Philadelphia.

21 Willats, S.M. (1987) *Lecture Notes on Fluid and Electrolyte Balance*, 32–49. Blackwell Scientific Publications, Oxford.

22 Michell, A.R. (1983) Diuretics and cardiovascular function. *Proceedings of the Association for Veterinary Clinical Pharmacology and Therapeutics* **7**, 19–26.

23 Gaskell, C.J. (1985) The urinary system. In: *Feline Medicine and Therapeutics*, 133–51. Chandler, E.A., Gaskell, C.J. & Hilbery, A.D.E. (eds). Blackwell Scientific Publications, Oxford.

24 Herrtage, M.E. (1983) Management of renal disease in veterinary practice. In: *Veterinary Nephrology*, 230–47. Hall, L.W. (ed). Heinemann, London.

25 Bush, B.M. (1984) Urinary system. In: *Canine Medicine and Therapeutics*, 406–41. Chandler, E.A., Sutton, J.B. & Thompson, D.J. (eds). Blackwell Scientific Publications, Oxford.

26 Finco, D.R., Barsanti, J.A. & Crowell, W.A. (1983) In: *Feline Medicine*, 363–410. Pratt, P.W. (ed). American Veterinary Publications Inc., Santa Barbara.

27 Cowgill, L.D. (1984) Diseases of the kidney. In: *Veterinary Internal Medicine* 2nd edn, 1793–1879. Ettinger, S.J. (ed). W.B. Saunders, Philadelphia.

28 Gordon, D. (1983) Principles of dialysis and renal transplantation. In: *Veterinary Nephrology*, 211–29. Hall, L.W. (ed). Heinemann, London.

29 Parker, H.R. (1984) Peritoneal dialysis and hemofiltration. *Canine Nephrology*, 723–53. Harwal, USA.

30 Clark, C.H. (1983) Fluid therapy. In: *Feline Medicine*, 31–59. Pratt, P.W. (ed). American Veterinary Publications Inc., Santa Barbara.

31 Barsanti, J.A. & Finco, D.R. (1984) Management of post renal uraemia. *Veterinary Clinics of North America: Small Animal Practice* **14**(1), 609–15.

32 Michell, A.R. (1979) Drugs and renal function. *Journal of Veterinary Pharmacology and Therapeutics* **2**, 5–20.

33 Selcer, B. (1982) Urinary tract trauma associated with pelvic trauma. *Journal of the American Animal Hospital Association* **19**, 785–93.

34 Wingfield, W.E. (1974) Lower urinary tract injuries associated with pelvic trauma. *Canine Practice* **1**, 25–8.

35 Crane, S.W. (1980) Evaluation and management of abdominal trauma in the dog and cat (Symposium on Trauma). *Veterinary Clinics of North America: Small Animal Practice* **10**(3), 655–89.

36 Burrows, C.F. & Bovee, K.C. (1974) Metabolic changes due to experimentally induced rupture of the canine urinary bladder. *American Journal of Veterinary Research* **35**, 1083–8.

37 Pascoe, R.R. (1971) Repair of a defect in the bladder of a foal. *Australian Veterinary Journal* **47**, 343–4.

38 Rooney, J.R. (1971) Rupture of the urinary bladder in the foal. *Veterinary Pathology* **8**, 445–51.

39 Richardson, D.W. & Kohn, C.W. (1983) Uroperitoneum in the foal. *Journal of the American Veterinary Medical Association* **182**, 267–71.

40 Surawicz, B. (1967) Relationship between electrocardiogram and electrolytes. *American Heart Journal* **73**, 814–34.

41 Cuddeford, D. (1988) Ovine urolithiasis. In: *Urolithiasis in Animals*, 143–52. Moreau, P. (ed). Proceedings of the 3rd Annual Symposium of ESVNU (European Society of Veterinary Nephrology and Urology). Intercongress, Barcelona.

42 O'Rourke, R.A. (1984) *The Heart and Renal Disease*, 52–5. Churchill Livingstone, New York.

Chapter 11 _____
Anaesthesia, surgery and fluid therapy

Introduction

It is difficult to be prescriptive about fluid therapy in association with surgery because even in the one species which has experienced massive numbers of surgical interventions with detailed monitoring of the consequences, namely man, great uncertainties remain. Comparable information from clinical cases, as opposed to experimental animals, is fragmentary for species of primary veterinary concern. We can, therefore, do little more than understand principles and apply them across the species, recognizing that important differences may exist.

There are a number of possible reasons to give fluids during or immediately after surgery:
1 To prevent or treat shock.
2 To treat dehydration and electrolyte losses.
3 To correct acidosis.
4 To maintain intravenous access.
5 To supply nutrients.
A number of fluids are frequently used: colloids, crystalloids, dextrose or dextrose–saline mixtures and blood or blood derivatives.

In order to maintain stable cardiovascular and renal function it is desirable that, as far as possible, recognizable deficits are corrected before surgery. Only potentially serious disturbances should be corrected during surgery. Other objectives, e.g. provision of maintenance requirements, should be postponed until recovery, indeed the animal may readily solve the problem by resumption of drinking and eating. Following surgery, if other aspects of the condition do not contraindicate oral fluids, they are likely to be well absorbed and appropriate.

The main indications for intravenous fluid therapy during surgery would therefore seem to be:
1 Correction of circulating volume.
2 Replacement of overt losses — haemorrhage, evaporation from wound surfaces, removal of fluids and electrolytes from or with damaged viscera or tissue.

What complicates the problem is that:

1 Anaesthesia and surgery both disturb the renal regulation of body fluids.

2 Surgery may trigger the normal metabolic response to trauma [1] which further interferes with regulation of ECF volume and composition.

3 There is considerable controversy as to the importance of concealed loss or sequestration of fluid into damaged tissues during surgery. The formation of such 'third space' clearly occurs, and may go beyond the immediate area of intervention particularly if there is shock or widespread underperfusion of tissues. Nevertheless, some estimates of its occurrence may have been exaggerated by technical problems including poor equilibration of 'markers' or their loss from ECF via damaged membranes rather than dilution by sequestered extravascular fluid. Not only is there uncertainty about the scale, frequency and importance of such concealed losses, there is even greater ambiguity about the extent to which renal salt and water retention are appropriate responses to deficits initiated by surgery or represent additional disturbances triggered by anaesthesia and surgery.

In the 1950s the work of Moore suggested that sodium and water retention was an obligatory response to surgical stress and that the restriction of sodium and water intake in the peri-operative period constituted rational therapy. This view was challenged by Shires [2] in the early 1960s; he postulated that the ECF volume decreased during major surgery due to internal redistribution of body fluids, probably through paralytic ileus or wound oedema. His suggestion was that fluid entered this 'third space' resulting in a true fluid deficit needing intravenous replacement with crystalloids. Many studies appeared to confirm Shires' views. A disproportionate deficit in plasma volume has been demonstrated in human patients undergoing extensive surgery together with a reduced ECF volume beyond that expected from blood loss alone. Other workers, however, have been unable to demonstrate any post-operative decrease in ECF and have criticized Shires' techniques. Equally, however, changes in the excretion of 'markers' used to measure body fluid compartments may have masked the occurrence of real deficits associated with surgery [2].

The practical questions which arise, therefore, are: other than to correct obvious losses and disturbances associated with the condition (e.g. gastric torsion) or the surgery (e.g. removal of major portions of gut or a distended uterus) when does surgery necessitate or justify fluid therapy? And if it is given, how important is it to maintain PCV (i.e. avoid haemodilution), and to protect plasma composition (notably Na, bicarbonate and K) as well as circulating volume. Colloids or electrolytes? Saline or Hartmann's? Dextrose or electrolytes? What rates or volumes are safe and reasonable?

The 'colloid versus crystalloid' controversy now centres frequently on issues relating to philosophy, side effects and economics. The arguments on both sides have been outlined in a number of reviews [3−6]. Following Shires' publications, fluid restriction, as advocated by Moore, gave way to fluid inundation and the widespread use of buffered or balanced electrolyte solutions. This prompted a joint editorial by both Moore and Shires urging moderation. Yet many current peri-operative regimens, especially in North America, appear to be dominated by the fear that renal failure and sudden post-operative hyperkalaemia may follow surgery unless relatively large volumes of electrolyte solutions are infused. It is more likely that a conservative approach modified according to the individual clinical case and the patient's response will result in a satisfactory outcome.

Normally, excess fluids are well tolerated in the absence of cardiac or pulmonary dysfunction and of sepsis. Trauma, which includes surgery, however, undermines the resistance to pulmonary oedema and both surgery and anaesthesia undermine the renal response to excess fluids. An understanding of these renal changes is central to rational decisions in this controversial area of fluid therapy.

Renal changes during anaesthesia and surgery

These have been reviewed in detail [7, 8] and vary with species and anaesthetic. Nevertheless, the reasons for the changes are direct effects of anaesthesia on renal function, interference with renal auto-regulation, cardiovascular responses affecting the kidneys (notably hypotension), effects mediated by renal nerves, and hormonal changes associated both with anaesthesia and surgery. Clinically, the patient responds to the combined influence of surgery and anaesthesia although each has separate effects. The character of the response is considerably influenced by any associated hypovolaemia or hypo-tension and, to a lesser extent, by prior sodium intake [8, 9].

The most striking effect, first observed in dogs in 1905, is post-operative urine retention [9]. This is only partly mediated by ADH and also reflects changes in GFR and solute load [10]. The rise in

ADH is particularly associated with abdominal surgery and specific stimuli include pain, stress, hypoxia and traction on abdominal viscera, apart from 'relevant' stimuli such as hypovolaemia and hypotension [11]. Although ADH may not be the only factor causing post-operative water retention, while plasma ADH is elevated the animal is less likely to satisfactorily excrete any excess water [10].

There is also an increase of aldosterone secretion which only lasts a few hours if patients are prevented from becoming hypovolaemic, but impairment of sodium excretion may nevertheless last for several days [12]. Anaesthesia also activates the renin−angiotensin system and this is especially marked in hypovolaemia and contributes to the decline in renal function [7]. Not surprisingly, the adverse effects of anaesthesia on renal function are greatly intensified not only by depth of anaesthesia but by concurrent dehydration [8].

The increase in ADH secretion associated with surgery can persist for one or several days and is not prevented by deliberate expansion of plasma volume by colloids; it may represent a response to, and protection against hypotension since ADH is also a powerful vasocon-strictor [9]. While both sodium and water may thus be retained for reasons unrelated to fluid balance, the general trend is for the water retention to be quantitatively more significant, i.e. for plasma Na^+ to fall. Indeed, observations in dogs and cats suggest that water retention may occur without sodium retention [13]. Moreover, a volume depleted animal with hyponatraemia has difficulty excreting any administered excess of water, not only because of ADH but because delivery of fluid to the loop, responsible for dilution of urine (Chapter 1), is reduced [14]. Any tendency towards hyponatraemia may be reinforced during hypovolaemia by the 'sick cell syndrome', i.e. failure of cellular sodium pumps to restrict sodium to the ECF as efficiently as normal [15]. In view of these multiple factors tending to lower plasma sodium concentration and to restrict excretion of excess water, there is little justification for administering water (i.e. 5% dextrose) parenterally during surgery. In a 20 kg animal with a plasma sodium concentration of 140 mmol/l, 1 litre of dextrose, in the presence of renal water retention, could well drop plasma Na^+ below 130 mmol/l. It is true that an animal's maintenance requirements of water and electrolytes are well represented by dilute electrolyte solutions made isotonic with dextrose (Chapter 12). But the period immediately surrounding surgery is no time to deal with maintenance requirements: circulating volume is the issue of concern and hyponatraemia is an unwanted complication, particularly in veterinary practice where plasma Na is seldom measured. Since the excretion of 'free water' may be restricted for several days after major surgery, excessive administration or consumption of water should be avoided during this period. Watch must also be kept, however, for any developing abnormal fluid loss or signs of dehydration.

All these considerations apply to animals with basically healthy kidneys. Unfortunately, animals with substantial loss of renal function are at particular risk because they may be asymptomatic with minimal changes in plasma biochemistry. Both anaesthesia and dehydration are likely to decompensate their renal function. It is all the more important, especially in older animals where the likelihood of renal dysfunction is greater, to monitor plasma urea or creatinine pre-operatively and to rectify dehydration, as far as possible, prior to surgery. Such animals are also more likely to have metabolic acidosis, and anaesthesia may well interfere with respiratory compensation, so intensifying the fall in plasma pH.

Horses under anaesthesia, especially with halothane, tend to react as though they are hypovolaemic and may develop substantial degrees of arterial hypotension. Rather than attempting to treat this with drugs to improve cardiac output or reduce peripheral vasodilatation, the infusion of 5−15 l/hour of lactated Ringer solution is usually effective in restoring both arterial pressure and tissue perfusion.

Therapeutic implications

During minor surgery or brief operations in healthy animals, fluid administration is unnecessary, adds expense and might even be detrimental. In general, animals should come to anaesthesia well hydrated and there should be no restriction on drinking beforehand except where animals are vomiting.

The main adverse effects of fluid therapy during surgery, provided rates are not excessive, would be haemodilution, dilutional acidosis and hyponatraemia. The arguments concerning crystalloids versus colloids have been discussed in Chapter 3. The fact that some degree of haemodilution improves oxygen delivery, by improved viscosity of blood and increased cardiac output, has also been emphasized (Chapter 4). The fear that tissue oxygenation and wound healing may be impaired seems exaggerated; at PCVs above 17−20%, wound Po_2 is independent of PCV [16]. Thus, risks from a reduced PCV through the use of parenteral fluids mainly arise in animals already compromised by cardiac (or respiratory) problems.

Concerning colloids versus crystalloids, the problem is not 'either/ or'; colloids provide a useful way of holding additional crystalloids in circulation [17] and this is particularly appropriate if 'third space' accumulation is considered a problem. Nevertheless, both pharmacological and financial constraints limit their use and, in general, 20 ml/kg is a maximum dose. Since the main purpose of fluid therapy during surgery is to protect ECF volume, especially circulating volume, solutions must contain plasma-like amounts of sodium. Dextrose (5%) is essentially a source of water (Chapter 3) and most of the water will end up in cells instead of ECF. Moreover, it tends to depress plasma sodium and, in so far as 'irrelevant' salt and water retention is a frequent complication of major surgery, the evidence suggests that water retention is the prominent effect, i.e. the outcome will be to predispose to hyponatraemia. Genuine volume depletion also predisposes to hyponatraemia (Chapter 2). Even if it is argued that surgery increases evaporative water loss, as it does, the animal is likely to more than compensate for this once it resumes drinking and, meanwhile, Hartmann's solution (Na = 131 mmol/l) effectively contains 10% free water compared with ECF (Na = 145 mmol/l). Thus, there is little to commend the use of dextrose solutions *during* surgery in the absence of hypoglycaemia. The main exception would be in advanced shock, especially endotoxin shock, but even there, replacement of circulating volume is the first priority. Addition of glucose may, however, be necessary but this is preferably decided in the light of a blood glucose reading, since the early stages of traumatic shock often cause hyperglycaemia (Chapter 4).

Since the common acid−base disturbance associated with shock and a number of conditions requiring surgery is metabolic acidosis [18], there is little justification for the routine use of bicarbonate-free solutions, e.g. Ringer's or saline, unless metabolic alkalosis has been diagnosed.

Conclusion

The conclusions, therefore, are that:

1 Where possible, deficits and disturbances should be corrected before anaesthesia and surgery.

2 Other than the correction of specific deficits and disturbances, e.g.

acidosis, shock, the precautionary use of fluid therapy should be restricted to Hartmann's or similar solutions and in amounts not exceeding 5−10 ml/kg/hour or 30−40 ml/kg. Smaller amounts of colloids may also be justifiable.

References

1 Michell, A.R. (1985) What is shock? *Journal of Small Animal Practice* **265**, 719−38.
2 Roberts, J.P., Roberts, J.D., Skinner, C., Illner, H., Canizaro, P.C. & Shires, G.T (1985) Extracellular fluid deficit following operations and its correction with Ringer's lactate. *Annals of Surgery* **202**, 1−8.
3 Shoemaker, W.C. & Hauser, C.J. (1979) Critique of crystalloid vs. colloid therapy in shock and shock lung. *Critical Care Medicine* **7**, 117−25.
4 Virgilio, R.W., Smith, D.E. & Zarins, C.K. (1979) Balanced electrolyte solutions: experimental and clinical studies. *Critical Care Medicine* **7**, 98−103.
5 Poole, G.V. Meredith, J.W., Pennell, T. & Mills, S.A. (1982) Comparison of colloids and crystalloids in resuscitation from haemorrhagic shock. *Surgery, Gynecology and Obstetrics* **154**, 577−86.
6 Haupt, M.T. (1986) Colloidal and crystalloid fluid resuscitation in shock associated with increased capillary permeability. In: *Albumin and the Systemic Circulation,* 86−100. Blauhut, B. & Lundsgaard-Hansen, P., (eds). Karger, Basel.
7 Mujais, S.K. (1986) Tansport and renal effects of general anaesthetics. *Seminars in Nephrology* **6**, 251−8.
8 Michell, A.R. (1981) Anaesthesia and the kidney. *Proceedings of the Association of Veterinary Anaesthetists of Great Britain & Ireland* **9**, 111−24.
9 Fieldman, N.R. (1988) The role of arginine vasopressin in the regulation of urinary output in the perioperative period. Master of Surgery Thesis, University of Cambridge.
10 Fieldman, N.R., Forsling, M.L. & Le Quesne, L.P. (1985) The effect of vasopressin on solute and water excretion during and after surgical operation. *Annals of Surgery* **201**, 383−90.
11 Haas, M. & Glick, S. (1978) Radioimmunoassayable plasma vasopressin associated with surgery. *Archives of Surgery* **113**, 597−600.
12 Le Quesne, L.P., Cochrane, J.P.S. & Fieldman, N.R. (1985) Fluid and electrolyte disturbances after trauma: the role of adrenocortical and pituitary hormones. *British Medical Bulletin* **41**, 212−17.
13 Hall, L.W. (1980) Preliminary investigations of the effects of injury on the body fluids of cats and dogs. *Journal of Small Animal Practice* **21**, 679−89.
14 Shapiro, J.I. & Anderson, R.J. (1987) Sodium depletion states. In: *Body Fluid Homeostasis,* 245−76. Brenner, B.M. & Stein, J.H. (eds). Churchill Livingstone, New York.
15 Illner, H. (1984) Changes in red blood cell transport in shock. In: *Shock and Related Topics,* 25−43. Shires, G.T. (ed). Churchill Livingstone, New York.
16 Hunt, T.K., Rabkin, J. & Van Smitten, K. (1986) Effects of edema and anemia on wound healing and infection. In: *Albumin and the Systemic Circulation,* 101−13. Blauhut, B. & Lundsgaard-Hansen, P. (eds). Karger, Basel.
17 Smith, J.A.R. & Norman, J.N. (1982) The fluid of choice for the resuscitation of severe shock. *British Journal of Surgery* **69**, 702−5.
18 Clark, J. & Walker, W.F. (1983) Acid−base problems in surgery. *World Journal of Surgery* **7**, 590−8.

Chapter 12

Metabolic and endocrine disturbances: parenteral nutrition

Introduction

So far, this book has considered:

1 Regulation and disturbances of body fluids (Chapters 1, 2, and 4).

2 Identification and correction of deficits; clinical and laboratory assessment, choice and composition of fluids, practicalities of parenteral therapy including transfusion (Chapters 3 and 5−8).

3 Oral rehydration and gastrointestinal disturbances (Chapter 9).

4 Particular problems posed by urinary dysfunction, anaesthesia and surgery (Chapters 10 and 11).

Throughout, the emphasis has been on water balance, major cations (Na and K) and acid−base disturbances. This chapter concerns itself more particularly with conditions demanding additional consideration of energy supply or provision of nitrogen (e.g. prolonged anorexia) or conditions interfering with glucose utilization (e.g. diabetes mellitus) together with some other conditions which precipitate a need for fluid therapy in the absence of obvious external losses. It thus takes the principles set out in earlier chapters and applies them to more complicated or less obvious patterns of disturbance.

Parenteral nutrition

General objectives

Maintenance therapy has been discussed already and is a component for consideration in any general scheme of fluid therapy. It comprises no more than parenteral provision of water, to compensate for inability to drink and of low concentrations of various electrolytes to make up for cessation of intake via food. Cats are especially sensitive to the metabolic effects of anorexia [1]. Total parenteral nutrition (TPN) confronts the full range of problems posed by prolonged inappetance or the need to avoid oral intake. It can be fairly comprehensive in its objectives, dealing with calories, amino acids, vitamins and trace elements, but it is neither simple nor inexpensive. Where inappetance, rather than a need to avoid oral intake, is the problem, tube-feeding with simple nutrient solutions or homogenates is preferable, though this may necessitate the placement of a pharyngostomy or nasogastric tube [1, 2] (Chapter 7).

Problems and practicalities

Relatively few solutions for parenteral nutrition have been specifically produced for animal use and we know comparatively little about the specific requirements associated with particular clinical conditions in species of major veterinary concern. In contrast, total parenteral nutrition in human medicine has become a refined science based on detailed study of a variety of specific problems in both infants and adults [3, 4]. But many of the relevant principles appear applicable certainly to dogs, probably to cats and perhaps, at least, to young herbivores. Indeed, it is now 40 years since the first successful use of extended periods of total parenteral nutrition and this was in dogs [5].

The main problems arise from the need for an extended period of sterile intravenous access, demanding careful supervision and much more meticulous technique than conventional fluid therapy. Nutrient solutions provide ideal media for bacterial proliferation and catheters are liable to encourage phlebitis and ultimately thrombosis or systemic infection. The problem is compounded where high concentrations of dextrose (e.g. 40%) are used as a calorie source because they are very irritant (and therefore need to be used in a major vein, e.g. the jugular, which provides rapid dilution) [6−8]. The root of this problem is that dextrose solutions provide 3.4 kcal/g [9] and, for example, an adult dog of 20 kg weight requires some 1200 kcal for full maintenance [5, 10]. The requisite 350 g of glucose, at 5%, occupy 7 l. Even at 40%, 0.9 l of dextrose are needed and, since infusion rates above 0.5 g/kg/hour cause glycosuria [5], the time involved would be some 35 hours. Over-rapid infusion of concentrated dextrose solutions also carries a risk of hyperglycaemia, especially when additional insulin is not given. Not surprisingly, one of the central themes of parenteral nutrition is the quest for alternative energy sources, e.g. lipid emulsions. Fortunately, even partial provision of calorie requirement may reduce catabolism [5] — except in the case of the metabolic response to trauma (Chapter 4) where even supranormal provision fails to suppress this complex endocrine response [11, 12). Trauma, in this context, includes major surgery [13].

Provision of amino acids also poses problems; excessive use of protein hydrolysates causes depression, emesis and even convulsions in dogs and cats and this is especially true of mixtures containing glutamic and aspartic acids, whereas glycine tends to prevent vomiting [1]. Excessive use of cationic amino acids (arginine, lysine, histidine) may cause metabolic acidosis [14]. Over-provision of nitrogen is likely to cause azotaemia [3]. Among the essential amino acids, dogs and cats are especially dependent on arginine for conversion of ammonia to urea; taurine is an essential amino acid for cats. [2]

Lipid emulsions can also have adverse effects, including interference with phagocyte function and induction of increased pulmonary vascular resistance, at least in infants; this may reflect provision of prostaglandin precursors [15]. They may also alter drop size and, therefore, the expected infusion rate [7].

The common electrolyte disturbances caused by i.v. feeding are hypokalaemia and hypophosphataemia, the latter especially associated with use of glucose as the sole calorie source. Its importance lies in an associated fall in red cell 2,3-DPG and ATP, leading to interference with liberation of oxygen from oxyhaemoglobin [3]. With extended parenteral nutrition, trace element deficits may become important, notably zinc, hence they are included in some commercial solutions. Since sterility is so important, it is generally preferable to use single solutions, rather than mix components. Where mixing is necessary it must be done in the cleanest possible surroundings, into an emptied sterile fluid container and with maximum precautions to avoid loss of sterility [16]. It is also preferable to provide nitrogen and calories concurrently but since these often involve separate solutions, this implies the use of two i.v. lines; while this is acceptable in human medicine the additional supervision, difficulty and risk is probably unacceptable in most veterinary practice.

Materials and requirements

The adult maintenance requirements of dogs and cats are approximately those shown in Table 12.1 [10].

Whatever the energy source, at least 10% of the calories should be provided as amino acids (including protein hydrolysates) except,

Table 12.1 Maintenance requirements of adult dogs and cats

Cats	all sizes	80 kcal/kg*
Dogs	10 kg	70 kcal/kg
	20 kg	60 kcal/kg
	30 kg	55 kcal/kg
	40 kg	50 kcal/kg
Water and electrolyte requirements [5]		*c.* 800 ml/1000 kcal
together with		25 mmol Na$^+$ (30 mmol/l)
		22 mmol K$^+$ (27 mmol/l)
		18 mmol/l Cl$^-$ (23 mmol/l) or more
		+15−25 mmol/l base (bicarbonate or precursor)

* 1 kcal = 4.2 kJ.

perhaps, in renal failure [5]. Here the maximum provision should be 0.3 g/kg/24 hours of a 5% amino acid solution, in the absence of specific information concerning the requirements of the uraemic dog [17]. Because of the risk of hyperglycaemia from over-rapid infusion, or of hypoglycaemia from sudden cessation (leaving high levels of endogenous insulin) changes in infusion rate must not be abrupt. Initiation and termination should be gradual (over a few hours) [2].

Alternative calorie sources have included fructose, sorbitol (which undergoes hepatic conversion to fructose) and ethyl alcohol (which provides more calories than glucose) none of which require insulin for utilization. Nevertheless, excess can cause lactic acidosis so glucose remains an essential component of parenteral nutrition [3, 4, 10] and lipids should comprise no more than half the calorie intake [2].

Intralipid is an emulsion of soya bean oil and contains essential fatty acids, phospholipids and glycerol. At 10 or 20% it provides approximately 1000 or 2000 kcal/l (4200 or 8400 kJ) (compared with 340/l in 10% dextrose). As well as calories this is a source of essential fatty acids. Soya bean oil emulsions are preferable to cotton seed oil emulsions, especially in dogs and cats [9, 10]. The high calorie content of lipids is useful where excess water is harmful (e.g. acute renal failure) but not in cases with severe hyperlipaemia or hepatic disease [3].

Nitrogen is provided as L amino acids or hydrolysates of proteins such as casein. The inclusion of arginine (or ornithine) is obligatory for cats and dogs [1]. 'Aminoplex 5' contains a mixture of amino acids, sorbitol, ethanol, nicotinamide and vitamin B$_6$ and provides 5 g of N_2 and 1000 kcal/l; an average cat would need up to 500 ml and a 10 kg dog about 800 ml [10]. Infusion rates up to about 100 ml/hour into the vena cava are acceptable, but slower rates are preferable. In animals with hepatic disease, branched-chain amino acids may be particularly valuable (e.g. leucine, isoleucine, valine) [3, 4].

Since parenteral nutrition involves slow extended infusions, the use of specifically designed pumps for rate control is ideal — but again, the cost implies a real investment in high quality intensive care. The balance between costs, and effectiveness remains an open question in veterinary parenteral nutrition since clinical experience with it is, as yet, relatively limited. Even in human medicine, the benefits may have been overestimated [4]. Nevertheless, for periods where oral intake needs to be avoided for several days or longer, there is no alternative; traditional measures such as use of 5–10% dextrose will be wholly inadequate.

In any species, the nutritional requirements are increased in young, pregnant, lactating or febrile animals. Thus in dogs between weaning and half growth, the calorie requirement is about double that of a full grown dog of similar weight [10]. The comparable figure in cats is about $\times$ 1.6. Table 12.2 shows the requirements suggested for parenteral nutrition in foals. Appropriate mixtures should provide 100–200 kcal from non-protein sources/g of nitrogen given (1 g nitrogen = 6.2 g protein). A foal can be kept on total parenteral nutrition (100 kcal/kg) for a week without weight loss; oral feeding is introduced during a further three days of TPN [19]. A number of formulations have been suggested for TPN in foals; some of these may be suitable for calves [20]. The cost and complexity of TPN for adult horses makes it preferable whenever possible to use specifically formulated oral mixtures, if necessary by nasogastric tube (stomach tube) [16].

Finally, it should be emphasized that even where total parenteral

Table 12.2 Requirements for parenteral nutrition in foals

Water	100 ml/kg
Calories	150 kcal/kg
Protein	3 g/kg
Na^+	@ 13 mmol/l
K^+	@ 30 mmol/l
Cl^-	@ 40 mmol/l
+ phosphate, calcium, magnesium and vitamins (based on [18])	

nutrition is not contemplated, a day of inadequate fluid intake or $2-3$ days of anorexia still justify the relatively simple techniques of maintenance therapy. In neonates where venous access is impractical, the use of warm solutions intraperitoneally, with sterile precautions, is the alternative. If the subcutaneous route is used it may be preferable to use a $50:50$ mixture of Hartmann's solution and 5% dextrose to reduce the initial loss of Na^+ from circulation into the subcutaneous pool (which is why maintenance solutions are not intended for subcutaneous use). If oral rehydration solutions (Chapter 9) are used in anorectic rather than diarrhoeic animals it must be recognized that they alone cannot provide sufficient calories, being primarily formulated to promote intestinal uptake of sodium and water.

Diabetes mellitus

Pathophysiology

From a fluid and electrolyte point of view, the key disturbances in a destabilized diabetic are hyperosmolarity, osmotic diuresis and, perhaps, metabolic acidosis and ketosis [5, 21]. The osmotic diuresis may lead to extracellular volume depletion and thus undermine renal function. The hyperosmolarity results not only from the glucose but the excess water loss characteristic of osmotic diuresis [21, 22]. Any associated vomiting intensifies the dehydration but is likely to lessen the acidosis (unless there is reflux of intestinal contents). Unfortunately, the degree of hyperglycaemia does not predict the severity of the acidosis so a measurement of TCO_2 is worthwhile, particularly because severe acidosis blocks the response to insulin.

The volume depletion certainly merits treatment but whether or not to treat the acidosis, is controversial since it should improve in the aftermath of insulin therapy, provided it is not too severe. Overtreatment could then lead to metabolic alkalosis (direct effect of bicarbonate) plus respiratory alkalosis (caused by sudden elevation of plasma and CSF P_{CO_2}; Chapter 2).

While the animal may initially be hyperkalaemic, it is likely to become hypokalaemic as the acidosis subsides and, above all, as insulin drives both glucose and potassium into cells. Plasma sodium concentration (though not routinely measured) may either rise, reflecting the increased renal water loss, or fall because it is diluted by the extra water held in plasma by the additional glucose.

A further complication may arise from hypophosphataemia since this tends to depress 2,3-DPG concentration in red cells and impede the release of oxygen. This provides another reason for caution in the use of bicarbonate; any alkalotic overshoot will further impede the release of oxygen from haemoglobin [23]. On the other hand, bicarbonate is preferable to lactate which is unlikely to be utilized in ketotic animals.

Therapeutic implications

Although the dehydration is hypertonic, hypotonic solutions are best avoided initially since volume replacement is the priority and sudden changes in osmolality are undesirable [24, 25]. Thus treatment comprises:

1 Initial rehydration with saline unless:

2 The acidosis is severe in which case additional bicarbonate is needed; 15 mmol/l or 1 mmol/kg body weight with re-evaluation of response and adjustment of any additional dosage accordingly.

3 Alternate use of 'normal' and 'half-normal' saline [24, 26].

4 Once urine output is clearly adequate and acidosis is not severe additional K^+, some preferably as phosphate, should be included; in humans hypokalaemia can cause death in diabetic ketoacidosis [24]. Most K^+ should be supplied as chloride.

A precipitate fall of blood glucose is dangerous and may necessitate the use of 5% dextrose if the concentration rapidly falls below 1.5 mmol/l [24, 26, 27].

Hyperinsulinism in the dog [26]

Pathophysiology

Insulin-secreting tumours of the beta-cells of the pancreas are only diagnosed when the excess insulin produced results in hypoglycaemia severe enough to cause collapsing episodes which often resemble 'epileptic fits'. Unlike epilepsy, however, these fits tend to be precipitated by exercise and can be ameliorated by increasing the frequency of feeding.

Therapeutic implications

There are two distinct phases relating to the management of fluid therapy in these cases. Before surgery there is a real risk of severe hypoglycaemic collapse if these animals are starved for any length of time and it is therefore essential to set up an i.v. infusion of dextrose saline (N/5 + 4.3%) pre-operatively and to continue this infusion intra-operatively and in the immediate post-operative period. Some workers [26] recommend the administration of more concentrated solutions of dextrose (10% or even 50%) but this has not been necessary in our experience.

During surgery there is a risk of shock which will require treatment (Chapter 4), particularly where the tumour is in the body of the pancreas and the difficulty of removing it increases the likelihood of haemorrhage. Subsequently, especially if anything more than a minor degree of dissection has been required, there is a real risk of pancreatitis developing. These dogs frequently develop persistent hyperglycaemia within 24 hours of surgery which persists for several days. This poses additional problems in that the intense thirst that such hyperglycaemia provokes can lead to the dogs drinking incessantly if they are allowed free access to water. The excessive drinking is usually followed by vomition and a vicious circle can be set up. It is preferable, therefore, to avoid giving anything more than minimal amounts of fluids orally for 2–3 days post-operatively and to maintain fluid and electrolyte balance intravenously. If severe pancreatitis develops post-operatively, additional fluid and electrolyte imbalances may develop which are discussed below.

Acute pancreatitis [2, 28–30]

Pathophysiological problems

While the precise aetiology remains a matter of debate, acute necrotizing pancreatitis is a well-recognized disease in small animals, especially dogs. It involves a massive release of proteolytic and lipolytic enzymes, together with vasoactive kinins. The outcome is the loss of large volumes of protein-rich fluid into the peritoneal cavity with rapid development of hypovolaemic and endotoxin shock. Vomiting and intestinal sequestration of fluid, as a result of ileus, further exacerbate the fluid losses. In addition, the release of myocardial depressant factor tends to reinforce the tendency towards shock (Chapter 4). Renal function may be severely depressed [28].

Therapeutic implications

The primary fluid and electrolyte disturbance is thus hypovolaemic shock and the ideal fluids are Hartmann's and plasma. The latter has the special virtue of antiprotease activity, helping to reduce formation of kinins and MDF [28]. Clinically, colloid solutions such as Haemaccel prove very useful in quickly correcting the hypovolaemia although in experimental canine pancreatitis artificial colloids were less satisfactory than crystalloids [31]. As usual with shock, high infusion rates (up to 90 ml/kg/hour) may be needed initially but careful monitoring is required as the release of vasoactive kinins may increase the risk of pulmonary oedema. While vomiting can be profuse, the predominant acid−base disturbance is usually metabolic acidosis. This can be severe and may require the administration of additional bicarbonate. Once the acidosis improves, hypokalaemia may occur and potassium supplementation may be required. Hypocalcaemia often accompanies acute pancreatitis but seldom causes symptoms and may reflect a fall in albumin (and thus bound calcium) rather than free, active calcium. The use of calcium gluconate is probably, therefore, an unnecessary precaution in the absence of symptoms. Administration of excess bicarbonate increases protein binding of calcium and thus increases the chances of symptomatic hypocalcaemia. If hypocalcaemia is a problem, calcium gluconate (10%) at 0.5−1 ml/kg body weight is infused slowly to effect. These animals are often hyperglycaemic and therefore glucose-containing solutions should be avoided.

Acute pancreatitis may be ameliorated by the administration of 'Trasylol', a kallikrein inhibitor which blocks the release of vasoactive kinins and MDF (Chapter 4) in the damaged pancreas but the use of corticosteroids is more controversial.

Acute pancreatitis is one of the few circumstances where the use of corticosteroids in shock might have adverse effects — though the position remains uncertain. There is experimental evidence that they may cause pancreatitis but also that they may improve experimentally-induced pancreatitis [30]. Other measures such as analgesics, peritoneal lavage, and anticholinergic treatment should also be considered but are beyond the scope of this book.

During recovery from pancreatitis, food restriction is necessary for several days, hence i.v. maintenance therapy and possibly parenteral nutrition are needed.

Hepatic disease [2, 32–35]

Pathophysiological problems

Liver disease presents as acute hepatocellular disease, chronic cirrhosis (in both cases, with or without jaundice) or, especially in young animals, as a porto-systemic shunt. Hepatic failure causes fluid and electrolyte loss through anorexia, vomiting and diarrhoea. It can also cause polydipsia and polyuria [39]. In addition, hypoalbuminaemia may increase the risk of a reduced circulating volume as well as causing oedema and ascites. There is also a strong tendency towards excessive renal retention of salt and particularly water (hence hyponatraemia) [37, 38]. Failure of reticuloendothelial and detoxifying functions may increase the risk of endotoxin shock. Hypoglycaemia is not a frequent problem except in severe cases of liver disease. Hypokalaemia may result from depressed food intake but is a particular problem in liver disease because any associated metabolic alkalosis (Chapter 2) tends to convert ammonium ions into free ammonia. This crosses cell membranes more easily, thus increasing the risk of ammonia intoxication [40]. The tendency towards hypokalaemia is increased by secondary hyperaldosteronism, which also exacerbates the tendency to sodium retention in chronic disease.

The central problem, therefore, is of an animal which may have fluid deficits caused by anorexia, vomiting or diarrhoea, which may become seriously hypovolaemic, and yet whose underlying condition tends towards excess retention of salt (oedema, ascites) and water, i.e. towards hyponatraemia despite sodium retention. The retained sodium, however, is mainly extravascular and does not, therefore, prevent the development of loss of *circulating* volume which is made all the more likely by severe hypoalbuminaemia. Iatrogenic dehydration and hyponatraemia may be caused by excessive use of diuretics to treat the oedema [41].

Therapeutic implications

Since metabolic alkalosis is potentially a serious complication in hepatic disease, volume replacement should be with saline or Ringer's (not lactated Ringer's). Lactated Ringer's solution is doubly inappropriate since any acidosis, if present, is likely to be lactic acidosis associated with depressed lactate utilization. Where animals with hepatic failure have severe acidosis, bicarbonate rather than lactate should be used but with great caution regarding both dose and rates. In the absence of acidosis or the presence of hypokalaemia, additional K^+ is advisable, up to 30 mmol/l. Where the main problem is anorexia, rather than overt loss of fluids and electrolytes, dextrose saline (4.3% + N/5) or other maintenance solutions may be needed but excess must be avoided because of the underlying tendency towards hyponatraemia. Glucose supplementation will not only prevent hypoglycaemia but help lower levels of ammonia in the central nervous system (CNS), thus ameliorating any encephalopathy. However, a note of caution must be added since occasionally some dogs with liver disease develop insulin-resistant hyperglycaemia following i.v. therapy with a glucose-containing fluid and this together with hypoprotein-aemia and sodium retention will result in the development of oedema.

Additional measures include the use of plasma in severe hypo-albuminaemia or parenteral nutrition (see above). Blood transfusion may be necessitated by anaemia but the blood should be fresh as storage reduces clotting factors and increases ammonia content. Reduction in prothrombin synthesis makes haemorrhage a serious problem in animals having hepatic disease and requiring surgery. Removal of large volumes of ascitic fluid by paracentesis may cause hypovolaemia and so may excessive use of diuretics. Hypoalbuminaemia reduces total calcium, rather than free calcium, but any metabolic alkalosis may increase the chance of symptomatic hypocalcaemia (see above).

Liver disease is often associated with hyperventilation and respiratory alkalosis, though the reasons remain unclear. Unfortunately, this leads to one of the situations where the diagnostic use of TCO_2 can be misleading, in the absence of a pH measurement. The renal response to respiratory alkalosis is to excrete bicarbonate (Chapter 2) and this may register, correctly, as a fall in TCO_2. In this case, however, the problem is an alkalosis, and bicarbonate therapy is not only inappropriate but contraindicated.

Finally, it must be emphasized that in liver disease with ascites or oedema a conflict of therapeutic priorities can arise. Generally, sodium restriction and mobilization of excess sodium (oedema or ascitic fluid) with diuretics is advised. Except with pure water loss (hypernatraemia), repair of circulating volume is the priority for fluid therapy. The paradox is that despite the general expansion of ECF volume in oedema or ascites, plasma volume is not necessarily expanded, indeed with the reduced production of albumin it is likely to be subnormal

[36, 37]. As in many states with reduced circulating volume, plasma sodium concentration is liable to fall (Chapter 2). Thus despite the presence of excess sodium in the ECF, the need to repair plasma volume imposes a need to use a solution of plasma-like sodium content, with or without a colloid. A certain degree of volume replacement requires a certain quantity of sodium and the use of hypotonic solutions 'to avoid excess sodium' simply provides excess water. It is, however, true that volume replacement requires much greater care to avoid overload than in a normal animal because excessive rates or doses will simply fuel the ascites or oedema. In severe cases ascitic fluid (a modified transudate) may prove a useful source of protein-rich fluid for reinfusion. The risk of overload may be heightened by the fact that hepatic failure is liable to severely decompensate renal function or precipitate an unusual form of acute renal failure (hepatorenal syndrome) [36]. The importance of this in veterinary medicine remains uncertain because there has been little awareness of the condition [34].

Addison's disease [26, 42] (see Chapter 6)

Pathophysiology

Adrenal cortical insufficiency can lead to defective secretion of both glucocorticoids and mineralocorticoids. The latter defect causes increased urinary loss of sodium and thus contraction of ECF volume, ultimately leading to shock. It also impedes renal excretion of potassium, predisposing the animal to hyperkalaemia. Glucocorticoids normally oppose both the release and renal effects of ADH (i.e. they reduce water reabsorption in the collecting duct) and in their absence water reabsorption continues despite the resulting depression of plasma osmolality. This, together with volume depletion, leads to hyponatraemia.

Therapeutic implications

Apart from corticosteroid therapy the prime consideration is restoration of circulating volume and relief of hyperkalaemia; both are likely to respond to normal saline which may be supplemented with 5% dextrose since there is often hypoglycaemia. The acid–base changes are unpredictable, especially in dogs since the condition is uncommon and there is a lack of published data from clinical cases. Vomiting or diarrhoea could produce metabolic alkalosis or acidosis. In humans the lack of aldosterone impedes urinary acidification and thus causes renal tubular acidosis [43]. If the same is true in dogs, and in view of the hyperkalaemia, a bicarbonate source should be included rather than using simply saline. Hartmann's would seem appropriate, despite its K content (which is low). In addition, Addisonian crisis can cause acute renal failure, and thus acidosis. Often these cases present as vomiting collapsed dogs, and the underlying acidosis may be severe (i.e. base deficits in the range $10-20$ mmol/l; Chapter 6). Measurements of total CO_2 and blood urea are thus helpful in deciding between saline and bicarbonate-containing solutions for correction of volume depletion.

Pyometritis

Pathophysiology

Pyometritis is a common disorder in middle-aged, entire bitches and is probably one of the most frequent conditions for which fluid therapy is required in veterinary practice.

Bitches become dehydrated because of the loss of secretions into the uterus; these secretions are protein and electrolyte-rich and their loss may not be immediately obvious unless there is a vaginal discharge. Polyuria is also a feature of this disease and results in further fluid loss. The cause may be an immune-mediated glomerular dysfunction, together with depression of the renal response to ADH [44, 45].

Classically, the animal exhibits polydipsia but intake is generally still less than output, and as the bitch's condition deteriorates and vomiting starts, then severe dehydration leading to hypovolaemic shock occurs very quickly. Laboratory investigations can be misleading in pyometritis for these dogs often have a degree of anaemia and hypoproteinaemia which gives a falsely low haematocrit. Thus, one can be misled into assuming that they are not dehydrated.

Therapeutic implications

It is vital to correct dehydration in these bitches otherwise, although they may survive the surgery initially, they will develop renal failure and die some weeks later. The dilemma faced by the surgeon is how long one should delay surgery by giving fluids first, since until the operation has been performed, the excessive losses will continue. The aim must be to correct the circulating volume deficit, at least, before inducing anaesthesia, so that a precipitous fall in cardiac output can be avoided and renal perfusion maintained. The rest of the calculated deficit, which is often as much as 100–150 ml/kg is then replaced more slowly during and after surgery (over a period of 6–12 hours). The nature of the losses incurred dictates that a balanced electrolyte solution such as Hartmann's should be given, with or without a colloid. Intravenous maintenance fluids may be required for several days post-operatively until the polyuria subsides and the dog is able and willing to drink again. It is especially important to monitor the volume of fluid drunk and the volume of urine produced since these dogs often do not maintain positive fluid balance initially, and are prone to develop renal failure.

Peracute coliform mastitis [46, 47]

Pathophysiology

Acute mastitis caused by *E. coli* is perhaps the classic cause of endotoxin shock in cows. It is a life-threatening disease which results from the proliferation of organisms and release of bacterial endotoxin (lipo-polysaccharide). The endotoxin is absorbed and causes systemic effects which are, in effect, those of endotoxin shock.

The onset of disease is rapid, with early signs of agalactia, shivering and, usually, fever. Later the rectal temperature may fall to normal or below. The udder is swollen (in later stages) and the secretion from the teat is initially watery and eventually serous. Collapse may be rapid, and treatment must be urgent and aggressive to allow other than a very poor prognosis.

The need for fluid therapy therefore results not only from loss of fluid into the damaged mammary gland but from the systemic effects of endotoxin. These may be considerably advanced before mammary changes are obvious. While there may be substantial loss of fluid within the affected mammary tissue this is offset by the onset of agalactia. If the animal is febrile its water losses are increased and there may also be profuse watery diarrhoea leading to obvious dehy-dration. The loss of water and electrolytes is exacerbated by cessation of eating and drinking. Even in the absence of visible signs of dehydration, however, the central problem remains the treatment of endotoxin shock.

Therapeutic implications

The real difficulty is one of scale; there is no evidence, weight for weight, that cattle need any less fluids or other medication than other species with endotoxaemia. The problem is that the cost of adequate treatment may be economically prohibitive. Thus 40–60 l may be needed in 24 hours; 20–30 l in the first 2–6 hours, 10 l in the first 20 minutes (with monitoring of pulse and respiratory sounds). The first 6 l should be given as rapidly as possible, and a further 6 l then given over the subsequent 30–40 minutes. In order to increase the rate of administration, two infusions may be given simultaneously into either jugular or mammary veins (preferably the former, since a large needle may result in a haematoma if used in the mammary vein). Fluid given intravenously should preferably be warmed by a heating coil placed in a bucket of warm water. The logistic problems of administration of large volumes of fluid require a suitably large-bore needle (14 gauge), large containers (preferably 5 l) and a modicum of patience. This is likely to be rewarded when response can be seen in reversal of some of the symptoms of shock, with a fall in heart rate, improved peripheral circulation and even a return to a standing position.

The choice of fluids will in most cows be restricted by economic considerations to simple electrolyte solutions, although colloidal plasma expanders are theoretically desirable. Most of this fluid should be Hartmann's lactated Ringer solution together with 5% glucose (isotonic) since endotoxin shock characteristically produces hypoglycaemia. The electrolytes available in large packs (3–5 l) are isotonic saline, glucose saline and Hartmann's solution. All are likely to be beneficial, although the alkalinizing activity of Hartmann's solution is helpful in countering the acidosis present in most cases. The use of 0.9% saline, while meeting the primary object of protecting ECF volume, fails to deal with acidosis which is usually a feature of shock, hence the preference for Hartmann's or a solution with 20–30 mmol/l of bicarbonate.

The use of intravenous soluble corticosteroids is problematical since the benefits (Chapter 4) are only associated with 'massive' or 'pharmacological' doses such as 30 mg/kg of methylprednisolone. The difficulty is that not only is this expensive, but the assumption that it is effective is essentially based on impressions gained from other species.

Antibiotics (preferably bactericidal) should be given by the intravenous route, with intramammary administration following stripping of the secretion. The chosen antibiotics should have a good anti-Gram-negative activity. Colistin (polymyxin E) and polymyxin B are interesting in that both are claimed to specifically inactivate Gram-negative endotoxin, although the evidence for clinical benefit from this activity is still lacking. Anti-inflammatories, both steroidal and non-steroidal anti-inflammatory drugs (e.g. flunixin meglumine) may be useful in reducing the acute inflammation, although these (like antibiotics) are likely to be of less importance than fluid therapy. Oral fluid therapy may be useful as an adjunct to intravenous fluid, particularly where the intravenous volumes given are limited. Simple isotonic salt solutions may be given by stomach tube and pump, or specifically formulated oral fluid replacers may be used where economically justified.

The use of 'home-made' parenteral solutions has been advocated where costs are otherwise prohibitive. The risks of this have been explained in Chapter 7 and they must be explained to the farmer in case of pyrogenic reactions or worse. If such a course is adopted, and having explained the risks, certain precautions are simple and inexpensive:

1 The use of a constant source of boiled mains water (i.e. the practice)
2 Weighing into sachets sodium chloride and bicarbonate as follows (the latter is liable to precipitate with unboiled hard water): sodium bicarbonate (25 g) and sodium chloride (67 g) dissolved in 10 l produces Na 145 mmol/l, Cl 115 mmol/l, HCO_3 30 mmol/l.

Even with boiled water, such a solution is a considerable risk and any justification is considerably reduced by the growing availability of commercial solutions in large-volume packs. The additional procedures required for 'home-preparation' of sterile fluids have been discussed by Corke [48].

Exercise-induced fluid and electrolyte losses in greyhounds

The racing greyhound is in a high state of training for the relatively brief but intensely strenuous exercise of racing. The fluid losses are therefore analagous with the human sprinter rather than with the endurance marathon runner. There is therefore a less clear need for specific replacement of electrolytes since sweating in the dog is insignificant in terms of heat regulation, while body temperature is largely maintained through panting. This will cause loss of water, but there will be relatively little accompanying loss of sodium or chloride through sweat, in contrast to the horse (see below).

The racing greyhound should be offered water to replace that lost through panting. The water may be in the form of an oral rehydration formulation in order to maximize absorption. However, in view of the minimal loss of electrolyte, this may be diluted $1:4$ in comparison with the isotonic strength used to replace losses in diarrhoea.

Exercise-induced dehydration in horses [49]

Pathophysiology

Two distinct types of endurance rides give rise to problems of fluid and electrolyte imbalances in horses. Short (3−10 km) but fast races in hot weather cause slight dehydration but because of a tendency to depletion of energy stores and a switch to anaerobic metabolism severe metabolic lactic acidosis develops. Generally, horses lose only around 2−10 l of water and 200−500 mmol Na^+ and 100−500 mmol K^+ and require only oral rehydration fluids with added potassium salts to make good the loss. Some horses may show an increase in plasma sodium after exercise, probably through increased absorption of gut fluids.

Protracted endurance rides of 80−100 km or so ridden at a slower speed (10−18 km/hour) present a different problem. Energy is normally provided by aerobic metabolism of both carbohydrates and fatty acids with minimal metabolic changes until these substrates are exhausted. Most rides occur in the summer and the severity of problems encountered depends on the environmental temperature and humidity and the speed at which the horses travel.

In a moderate climate, such as is generally prevalent in the UK, horses subjected to an 80 km ride lose water equivalent to about 7% of their body weight (i.e. around 35 l) of which 6 l is lost from the plasma. As well as mixed loss of water and electrolytes in sweat, pure water loss from the respiratory tract is important and offsets the osmotic effect of the hypertonic losses in equine sweat [50]. Electrolyte losses consist of sodium, potassium and particularly chloride, and tend to be exacerbated in hot conditions as the horses sweat profusely and equine sweat is rich in K^+ and Cl^- ions. The horses may therefore become hyponatraemic, hypokalaemic and hypochloraemic. These changes will be exacerbated by immediate consumption of excessive quantities of water. Endurance horses become haemoconcentrated (PCV may rise to 60% or more) and because of the loss of chloride ions, develop a metabolic alkalosis.

Calcium losses in sweat and the shift to the unionized form provoked by the metabolic alkalosis produces a tendency to hypocalcaemia and the development of neuromuscular spasms including synchronous diaphragmatic flutter. Magnesium losses in sweat also predispose to hypomagnesaemic tetany in severe cases. In addition, exhaustion of glycogen stores results in hypoglycaemia and an increase in free fatty acid (FFA) concentration.

Therapeutic implications

Most horses will respond to rest, cooling water and food, but sometimes horses are so severely affected that they require more active therapy. Severely affected animals require the intravenous administration of an ECF expanding solution such as Hartmann's or 'normal' saline. Potassium should be added at around 10 mmol/l and dextrose will also be beneficial. Approximately 10−20 l given i.v. over 1 hour (4 l 5% dextrose and 16 l Hartmann's) are usually enough to improve the animal's condition sufficiently to allow full rehydration via orally administered fluids given, if necessary, by stomach tube. In extreme exhaustion horses may require 50−100 g/hour of dextrose in their i.v. fluids to correct hypoglycaemia. Horses exhibiting signs of synchronous diaphragmatic flutter and/or signs of ileus should be given calcium, added to the i.v. fluids at the rate of 100−300 ml 10−20% calcium borogluconate, given slowly to effect.

Occasionally, horses go on to develop exertional rhabdomyolysis a few days after an endurance ride. They are often animals which, although severely affected by the ride, received no fluid replacement therapy at the end of the ride. These horses tend to remain depressed and inappetant and then develop muscle stiffness, myoglobinaemia/uria, ileus and often laminitis. Treatment must consist of limiting further muscle damage, correcting fluid and electrolyte deficits and relieving discomfort. Non-steroidal anti-inflammatory drugs, corticosteroids and i.v. fluids are all indicated.

Prophylactic measures which may help prevent the onset of exertional rhabdomyolysis in those animals at risk include dantrolene sodium and vitamin E and selenium. Active cooling of hyperthermic horses at the end of a ride will also help reduce deleterious changes.

Fluid therapy has also been used in the treatment of equine anhidrosis (i.e. inadequate sweating response during exertion in hot climates) but its effectiveness is dubious [51].

Exertional myopathy (myoglobinuria, azoturia)

Pathophysiology

While exertional myopathy is seen in horses and dogs, much of our knowledge of the underlying problems is based on research directed towards a very similar condition in human athletes [52]. Muscle damage caused by extensive trauma is also a classic cause of acute renal failure in humans. The renal effects are determined not just by the amount of myoglobin released but by the concentration reached in renal tubules, hence the importance of diuresis. It is likely that the harmful effect of acidic urine is to cause myoglobin to dissociate into nephrotoxic products. The other 'product' of extensive muscle damage is potassium and both diuresis and alkalinization will protect against hyperkalaemia. The actual cause of the muscle damage appears to be any process interfering with delivery, storage or utilization of energy by muscle cells, including fasting, fever and viral influenza [52]. It is worth emphasizing that intracellular potassium deficits seriously impair energy metabolism and that potassium deficiency may also impede muscle blood flow; both these effects will predispose to rhabdomyolysis (muscle breakdown). Once it occurs, hyperkalaemia becomes a problem, despite any underlying potassium deficits.

Therapeutic implications

In this condition fluid therapy is used to protect the kidney rather than circulating volume or plasma composition. The risk is that myoglobin, a protein small enough to enter urine, will cause damage to renal tubules and precipitate acute renal failure [36]. This risk is greatest at low urine pH and high urine concentrations [53], hence the priority is to secure a brisk diuresis with a weakly acidic or alkaline urine. It is true that in horses there is some fluid loss through sweating associated with pain but this is not the reason for giving fluids. Where the precipitating exertion is severe, deficits may be added and, as in any acute renal failure, there is a risk of metabolic acidosis, though recent evidence suggests that a slight metabolic alkalosis is more usual [54, 55]. Since lactic acid may be involved in the pathogenesis, bicarbonate, rather than lactate, is generally preferred for treatment. Even in the absence of acidosis concentrations up to 30 mmol/l are reasonable in i.v. fluids since this is little more than normally present in plasma. Doses as low as 1 mg/kg $NaHCO_3$ [56] seem pointless since this is 5 mmol of bicarbonate in a 450 kg horse.

Lactic acidosis due to excess carbohydrate [57–59]

Engorgement on grain or excess of any other source of readily fermentable carbohydrate leads, through fermentation, to metabolic acidosis in herbivores, particularly cattle and horses. In particular, it leads to lactic acidosis which classically occurs [60] as:

Type A: with an apparent cause of hypoxia (shock, etc.)

Type B: no apparent hypoxia.

This condition is, therefore, a type B lactic acidosis caused by excess production whereas diabetes mellitus, also a type B acidosis, like that of bovine or ovine acetonaemia, is particularly characterized by defective lactate utilization. In the absence of uraemia or ketonaemia increased anion gap is strongly suggestive of lactic acidosis [61]. While the link between metabolic acidosis and hyperkalaemia may be controversial (at least in dogs: Chapter 2) it is generally suggested that metabolic acidosis due to organic acids is less likely to cause hyperkalaemia [62].

In ruminal acidosis, the fermentation not only produces acid but an increased osmotic concentration of breakdown solutes and this leads to accumulation of fluid within the rumen. In addition, gas production causes ruminal distension and impedes venous return. These factors may impair hepatic perfusion and thus superimpose poorer lactate utilization on the primary excess production. Although carbohydrate engorgement is the classical cause, any change in diet which alters the ruminal flora towards organisms (such as streptococci) which produce lactic acid from starch or glucose is a potential cause. The ruminal stasis which accompanies the condition mainly results from volatile fatty acid accumulation. Ultimately ruminal acidosis causes shock, potentially endotoxin shock, and lactic acidosis (metabolic acidosis) as the main problems. Intravenous saline and bicarbonate are thus appropriate but care should be taken to monitor progress and avoid excess bicarbonate because its potential adverse effects cause particular concern in lactic acidosis [63]. In theory, a mixture of bicarbonate and acetate may be preferable since lactate itself is clearly inappropriate in lactic acidosis. (Recent experiments in dogs suggest that a mixture of sodium carbonate and bicarbonate may be a good treatment for lactic acidosis; this is related to a specific model of type A, so further research is needed, even in dogs [64].) A conventional regimen [58] is 5 l of 5% sodium bicarbonate in the first 30 minutes for a 450 kg animal (7 mmol/kg approx.). This is followed up during the next 6−12 hours with 150 ml/kg of isotonic sodium bicarbonate. This is 23 mmol/kg and with such a high dose TCO_2 monitoring or more detailed acid−base evaluation is desirable during this period. Obviously, fluid therapy is only one aspect of the management of this condition but, especially in acute cases, it is a key factor in survival.

The condition in horses, from a fluid and electrolyte viewpoint, is fundamentally similar but overshadowed by the complications arising from extreme gastric dilatation. An important difference, however, is that much less lactic acid is absorbed and the lactic acidosis is much less severe, indeed aspiration of gastric contents may lead to metabolic alkalosis [65]. There may also be severe diarrhoea. The emphasis, therefore, is on restoration of circulating volume. Important complications of this condition are laminitis and gastric rupture which may make it rapidly fatal as a result of shock.

References

1 Clark, C.H. (1983) Fluid Therapy. In: *Feline Medicine*, 31−59. Pratt, P.W. (ed). American Veterinary Publications Inc., Santa Barbara.

2 Lewis, L.D., Morris, M.L. & Hand, M.S. (1987) *Small Animal Clinical Nutrition III*, 1:13−14; 5:1−43; 7:17−22; 7:52−58. Mark Morris Associates, Topeka.

3 Lee, H.A., Heatley, R.V. & Tredree, R. (1987) Practical aspects of intravenous feeding. In: *Clinical Nutrition in Gastroenterology*, 85−96; 116−29. Heatley, R.V., Losowsky, & Kelleker, J. (eds). Churchill Livingstone, Edinburgh.

4 Lee, H.A. (1974) Intravenous nutrition. *British Journal of Hospital Medicine* **11**, 719−24.

5 Michell, A.R. (1979) The physiological basis of fluid therapy in small animals. *Veterinary Record* **104**, 542−8.

6 Spurlock, S.L. & Spurlock, G.H. (1986) Considerations in catheter selection and maintenance in large animal species. In: *The Application of Intensive Care Therapies and Parenteral Nutrition in Large Animal Medicine*, 31−5. Rossdale, P.D. (ed). Travenol, Deerfield, Illinois.

7 Willatts, S.M. (1987) *Lecture Notes on Fluid and Electrolyte Balance*, 254−82. Blackwell Scientific Publications, Oxford.

8 Yoxall, A.T. & Hird, J.F.R. (1980) *Physiological Basis of Small Animal Medicine*, 127−78. Blackwell Scientific Publications, Oxford.

9 Kopple, J.B. & Blumenkrantz, M.J. (1980) Total parenteral nutrition and parenteral fluid therapy. In: *Clinical Disorders of Fluid and Electrolyte Metabolism*, 460−88. Maxwell, M.H. & Kleeman, C.R. (eds). McGraw Hill, New York.

10 Hall, L.W. (1982) Fluid therapy and intravenous nutrition. In: *Dog and Cat Nutrition*, 97−104. Edney, A.T.B. (ed). Pergamon, Oxford.

11 Michell, A.R. (1974) The metabolic consequences of trauma. *Journal of Small Animal Practice* **15**, 279−91.

12 Aulick, L.H. & Wilmore, D.W. (1983) Hypermetabolism in trauma. In: *Mammalian Thermogenesis*, 259−303. Girardier, L. & Stock, M.J. (eds). Chapman & Hall, London.

13 Muir, W.M. & DiBartola, S.P. (1983) Fluid Therapy. In: *Current Veterinary Therapy VIII*, 28−40. Kirk, R.W. (ed). W.B. Saunders, Philadelphia.

14 Clark, J. & Walker, W.F. (1983) Acid−base problems in surgery. *World Journal of Surgery* **7**, 590−8.

15 Lloyd, T.R. & Boucek, M.M. (1986) Effect of intralipid on the neonatal pulmonary bed. *Journal of Pediatrics* **108**, 130−3.

16 Naylor, J.M. & Freeman, D.E. (1987) Nutrition of the sick horse. In: *Current Therapy in Equine Medicine II*, 424−6. Robinson, N.E. (ed). W.B. Saunders, Philadelphia.

17 Finco, D.R. & Barsanti, J.A. (1983) Parenteral nutrition during a uraemic crisis. In: *Current Veterinary Therapy VIII*, 994−6. Kirk, R.W. (ed). W.B. Saunders, Philadelphia.

18 Mansmann, R., McAllister, E. and Pratt, P. (1982) *Equine Medicine and Surgery*, 310−316. American Veterinary Publications Inc., Santa Barbara.

19 Baker, J.C. & Ames, T.R. (1987) Total parenteral nutritional therapy of a foal with diarrhoea. *Equine Veterinary Journal* **19**, 342−4.

20 Hansen, T.O. (1986) Parenteral nutrition for foals and calves. In: *The Application of Intensive Care Therapies and Parenteral Nutrition in Large Animal Medicine*, 36−8. Rossdale, P.D. (ed). Travenol, Deesfield, Illinois.

21 Michell, A.R. (1979) Fluid therapy: some specific applications to medical conditions in small animals. *Veterinary Record* **104**, 572−5.

22 Michell, A.R. (1979) Drugs and renal function. *Journal of Veterinary Pharmacology and Therapeutics* **2**, 5−20.

23 Hoenig, M. (1986) Diabetic ketoacidosis. In: *Current Veterinary Therapy IX*, 987−91. Kirk, R.W. (ed). W.B. Saunders, Philadelphia.

24 Carroll, H.J. & Oh, M.S. (1978) Disturbances in acid−base balance. In: *Water, Electrolyte and Acid−Base Metabolism*, 216−305. Lippincott, Philadelphia.

25 Schade, D.S. & Eaton, R.P. (1983) Diabetic ketoacidosis — pathogenesis, prevention and therapy. *Clinical Endocrinology and Metabolism* **12**, 321−38.

26 Bush, B.M. (1984) The endocrine system. In: *Canine Medicine and Therapeutics*, 206−43. Chandler, E.A., Sutton, J.B. & Thompson, D.J. (eds). Blackwell Scientific Publications, Oxford.

27 Gruffyd-Jones, T. & Orr, C.M. (1985) The endocrine system. In: *Feline Medicine and Therapeutics*, 237−47. Chandler, E.S., Gaskell, C.J. & Hilbery, A.D.E. (eds). Blackwell Scientific Publications, Oxford.

28 Levy, M., Geller, R. & Hymovitch, S. (1986) Renal failure in dogs with experimental acute pancreatitis; role of hypovolaemia. *American Journal of Physiology* **251F**, 969−77.

29 Twedt, D.C. & Grauer, G.F. (1982) Fluid therapy for gastrointestinal, pancreatic and hepatic disorders. *Veterinary Clinics of North America: Small Animal Practice* **12**, 63−87.

30 Hardy, R.M. (1980) Inflammatory pancreatic disease. In: *Veterinary Gastroenterology*, 621−36. Anderson, N.V. (ed). Lea & Febiger, Philadelphia.

31 Martin, D.T. (1984) Crystalloid vs. colloid resuscitation in pancreatitis. *Surgery Gynecology and Obstetrics* **159**, 445−9.

32 Manderino, D.M. & De Vries, J. (1985) Hepatic encephalopathy. *Modern Veterinary Practice* **66**, 975−84.

33 Tams, T.R. (1985) Hepatic encephalopathy. *Veterinary Clinics of North America: Small Animal Practice* **15**, 177−95.

34 Grauer, G.F. & Rhett Nichols, C.E. (1985) Ascites, renal abnormalities and electrolyte and acid−base disorders associated with liver disease. *Veterinary Clinics of North America: Small Animal Practice* **15**, 197−214.

35 Wilkinson, S.P. (1984) Ascites, diuretics and surgery. In: *Liver*, 308−30. Williams, R. & Maddrey, W.C. (eds). Butterworths, London.

36 Michell, A.R. (1983) Abnormalities of renal function. In: *Veterinary Nephrology*, 189−210. Hall, L.W. (ed). Heinemann, London.

37 Epstein, M. (1987) Pathogenesis of sodium retention in liver disease. In: *Body Fluid Homeostasis*, 299−333. Brenner, B.M. & Stein, J.H. (eds). Churchill Livingstone, New York.

38 Michell, A.R. (1989) Regulation of salt and water balance (Waltham Symposium 1988). *Journal of Small Animal Practice*. In Press.

39 Bush, B.M. (1988) Polyuria and polydipsia. In: *Renal Disease in Dogs and Cats*, 48−74. Michell, A.R. (ed). Blackwell Scientific Publications, Oxford.

40 Michell, A.R. (1979) Biochemistry and behaviour: systemic aspects of neurological disturbances. *Journal of Small Animal Practice* **20**, 645−59.

41 Michell, A.R. (1988) Diuretics and cardiovascular disease. *Journal of Veterinary Pharmacology and Therapeutics* **11**, 246−53.

42 Lavelle, R.B. & Yoxall, A.T. (1980) The adrenal glands. In: *Physiological Basis of Small Animal Medicine*, 39−68. Yoxall, A.T. & Hird, J.F.R. (eds) Blackwell Scientific Publications, Oxford.

43 Walmsley, R.N. & Guerin, M.D. (1984) *Disorders of Fluid and Electrolyte Balance*, 40−1; 63; 201−2; 253−4. Wright, Bristol.

44 Bovee, K.C. (1984) *Canine Nephrology*, 327−38. Harwal, Philadelphia.

45 Obel, A., Nicander, L. & Asheim, A. (1964) A reversible mixed membrane proliferative glomerulo-nephritis. *Acta Veterinaria Scandinavica* **65**, 146.

46 Jackson, E. & Bramley, J. (1983) Coliform mastitis. *In Practice* **5**, 135−46.

47 Blood, D.C., Radostits, O.M. & Henderson, J.A. (1983) *Veterinary Medicine*, 471−6. Bailliere, London.

48 Corke, M.J. (1988) Economical preparation of fluids for intravenous use in cattle practice. *Veterinary Record* **122**, 305−7.

49 Rose, R.J., Carlson, G.P. & Warner, A. (1987) In: *Current Therapy in Equine Medicine II*, 187−8; 479−90. Robinson, N.E. (ed). W.B. Saunders, Philadelphia.

50 Kerr, M.G. (1986) Biochemical and physiological aspects of endurance exercise in the horse. PhD Thesis, University of Glasgow.

51 Warner, A. (1985) Equine anhidrosis. In: *Equine Medicine and Surgery in Practice*, 35−9. Whitlock, R.H. (ed). Veterinary Learning Systems, Lawrenceville, New Jersey.

52 Knochel, J.P. (1981) Rhabdomyolysis and myoglobinuria. *Seminars in Nephrology* **1**, 75−86.

53 Dubrow, A. & Flamanbaum, W. (1988) Acute renal failure associated with myoglobinuria. In: *Acute Renal Failure*, 279−95. Brenner, B.M. & Lazarus, J.M. (eds). Churchill Livingstone, New York.

54 White, K.K. (1983) Exertional myopathy. In: *Current Therapy in Equine Medicine*, 101−4. Robinson, N.E. (ed). W.B. Saunders, Philadelphia.

55 Hodgson, D.R. (1987) Exertional rhabdomyolysis. In: *Current Therapy in Equine Medicine*, 487−90. Robinson, N.E. (ed). W.B. Saunders, Philadelphia.

56 Mansmann, R., McAllister, E. & Pratt, P. (1982) In: *Equine Medicine and Surgery*, 3rd edn, 940−3. American Veterinary Publications Inc., Santa Barbara.

57 Michell, A.R. (1988) Metabolic acidosis. *In Practice*. In Press.

58 Blood, D.C., Radostits, O.M. & Henderson, J.A. (1983) *Veterinary Medicine*, 6th edition, 164−7; 221−7, Bailliere, London.

59 Whitlock, R.H. & Kronfeld, D.S. (1980) Ruminal lactic acidosis. In: *Veterinary Gastroenterology*, 238; 397−401. Anderson, N.V. (ed). Lea & Febiger, Philadelphia.

60 Narins, R.G. & Gardner, L.B. (1981) Simple acid−base disturbances. *Medical Clinics of North America* **65**, 321−46.

61 Relman, A.S. (1978) Lactic acidosis. In: *Acid−Base and Potassium Homeostasis*, 65−100. Brenner, B.M. & Stein, J.H. (eds). Churchill Livingstone, New York.

62 Cohen, J.J. & Kassirer, J.P. (1982) Metabolic acidosis. *Acid Base*, 121−6. Little Brown & Co., Boston.

63 Park, R. & Arieff, A.I. (1983) Lactic acidosis: current concepts. *Clinical Endocrinology and Metabolism* **12**, 339−58.

64 Bersin, R.M. & Arieff, A.I. (1987) Metabolic and cardiac effects of carbicarb v. sodium bicarbonate in dogs with hypoxic lactic acidosis. *Proceedings of the International Congress on Nephrology X*, London, 106.

65 Carter, G.K. (1987) Gastric diseases. In: *Current Therapy in Equine Medicine* (2nd edn), 41−4. Robinson, N.E. (ed). W.B. Saunders, Philadelphia.

Appendix I
UK sources for catheters

The following is not intended to be a comprehensive list of catheters or suppliers nor an endorsement of these as opposed to other catheters or suppliers. It is simply to help practitioners find initial contacts if they wish to explore some of the techniques discussed in the main text (Chapter 7).

These catheters (and others) can usually be obtained through veterinary wholesale suppliers and this can avoid the need to order large numbers (as often required by manufacturers or main suppliers).

Deseret Medical Inc.
Products include E−Z Caths, Angiocaths. (Wide variety of lengths and diameters available.)

British suppliers:
>   Becton Dickenson
>   Between Towns Road
>   Cowley
>   Oxford OX4 3LY

Abbott Laboratories Ltd
Products include Abbocaths, Drum Reel catheter.
>   Hospital Product Division
>   Queenborough
>   Kent ME11 5EL

Portex
Products include Miniven, infusion coils.

British suppliers:
>   Arnolds Veterinary Products Ltd
>   Cartmel Drive
>   Harlescott
>   Shrewsbury
>   Salop SY1 3BT

Critikon
Products include Cathlon i.v.

Broadlands
Sunninghill
Ascot
Berkshire SL5 9JN

Suppliers include:
    Veterinary Drug Company PLC
    Common Road
    Dunnington
    York
    YO1 5RU

Braunule
Suppliers include:
    Southern Veterinary Services Ltd
    137 Malling Street
    Lewes
    East Sussex BN7 2RB

Vygon UK Ltd
Products include Intraflon i.v. cannulae.

British suppliers:
    Benkat Instruments
    8 Pelham Street
    Ilkeston
    Derbyshire DE7 8AR

Appendix II
Representative normal values

These are merely meant as a broad guide; normal ranges in any laboratory should be based on its own validated and quality controlled techniques, moreover for fluid therapy the most important aspect is response to therapy in serial measurements.

	Cats	Dogs	Horses	Cattle	Calves
Haematology					
Haemoglobin (g/dl)	12	15	15	12	12
PCV (%) (ml/dl)	35	46	42	35	36
RBC (10^{12}/l)	7.5	7.0	9.5	7.5	
MCV (fl)	47	70	46	50	
MCH (pg/RBC)	15	22.0	16	14	
MCHC (g/dl)	33	34	34	33	
Biochemistry (mmol/l plasma)					
Na	152	147	140	142	138
K	4.7	4.6	3.8[a]	4.9	5.3
Cl	120[b]	110	105	105	90
pH (pH units: blood)	7.42[c]	7.42[c]	7.42[c]	7.42[c]	7.42[c]
HCO_3	19	22	28	26	25[d]
Urea	8.3[e]	6.0	6.0[e]	6.0	4.3
Creatinine (μmol/l)	90[f]	110[f]	135	140	105
Glucose (plasma)[g]	5.2	4.8	4.9	3.2	5.4
Total protein (g/l)	70	65	70	70	65
Albumin (g/l)	30	30	33	34	26

[a] May be as low as 2.5. [b] May be up to 140. [c] Very variable in venous samples. [d] TCO_2 in whole venous blood by Harleco. [e] Up to 15 in some individuals. [f] Up to 150.
[g] Fasting: variable.
These values are based on:

1 Blood, D.C., Radostits, O.M. & Henderson, J.A. (1983) *Veterinary Medicine* (6th edn), Baillière Tindall, London.
2 Kerr, M.G. (1988) *Veterinary Laboratory Medicine*. Blackwell Scientific Publications, Oxford.
3 Short, C.E. (1987) *Principles and Practice of Veterinary Anaesthesia*. Williams & Wilkins, Baltimore.
4 Groutides, C.P. (1988) Fluid, electrolyte and acid–base balance in diarrhoeic calves. PhD Thesis, University of London.

Appendix III
Veterinary parenteral solutions

At the time of going to press, the following solutions have been specifically licensed for use in animals under UK legislation. A much wider range is licensed for use in humans (see Table 3.1).

1 Hartmann's
Isolec*: 5l packs for large animals (cattle, calves, horses);
Aqupharm† No. 11 for dogs and cats.

2 Maintenance solutions
Aqupharm No. 18 for dogs and cats;
Duphalyte‡ for horses, cattle, pigs, dogs and cats.

3 Darrow's
Aqupharm No. 10 for dogs and cats.

4 Ringer's
Aqupharm No. 9 for dogs and cats.

5 Saline (0.9%)
Aqupharm No. 1 for dogs and cats.

6 Glucose (5%) Saline (0.9%)
Aqupharm No. 3 for dogs and cats.

7 Glucose (5%)
Aqupharm No. 6 for dogs and cats.

* Ivex Pharmaceuticals Ltd, Larne, Northern Ireland.
† Animalcare Ltd, Common Road, Dunnington, York YO1 5RU.
‡ Duphar Veterinary Ltd, Solvay House, Southampton SO3 4QH.

Index _____